fP

Also by Brenda Watson, C.N.C.

The H.O.P.E. Formula: The Ultimate Health Secret
Essential Cleansing for Perfect Health
Gut Solutions: Natural Solutions to Your Digestive Problems
Renew Your Life: Improved Digestion and Detoxification
The Detox Strategy: Vibrant Health in 5 Easy Steps

THE Fiber 35 Diet

Nature's Weight Loss Secret

Brenda Watson, C.N.C.
with Leonard Smith, M.D.

Free Press
New York London Toronto Sydney

*f*P

FREE PRESS
A Division of Simon & Schuster, Inc.
1230 Avenue of the Americas
New York, NY 10020

FREE PRESS and colophon are trademarks
of Simon & Schuster, Inc.

For information regarding special discounts for bulk purchases,
please contact Simon & Schuster Special Sales at 1-800-456-6798
or business@simonandschuster.com

Art Direction: michael black / BLACK SUN®
Design: Jason Oakman

The Library of Congress catalogued the Free Press hardcover as follows:

Watson, Brenda
The fiber35 diet : nature's weight loss secret / Brenda Watson with Leonard Smith.
p. cm.
Includes bibliographical references (pp. 275–285) and indexes.
1. High-fiber diet. 2. High-carbohydrate diet. 3. Low-fat diet. 4. Naturopathy. 5. Self-care—Health.
I. Smith, Leonard, 1942—. II. Title.
RM237.6.F5343   2007
613.2'63—dc22   2006100636
Manufactured in the United States of America

10 9 8 7 6 5 4 3 2 1

ISBN-13: 978-1-4165-4718-1
ISBN-10: 1-4165-4718-5
ISBN-13: 978-1-4165-6009-8 (pbk)
ISBN-10: 1-4165-6009-2 (pbk)

For my mother, Mary;
at ninety years old you are an inspiration to us all.

And for my granddaughter, Wednesday;
an eight-year-old endless ray of sunshine

Contents

THE Fiber 35 Diet

THE FIBER35 DIET— NATURE'S WEIGHT LOSS SECRET

Research shows that in the United States alone, consumers spend roughly $30 billion annually trying to lose weight or prevent weight gain, with an estimated $1 billion to $2 billion spent on weight loss programs.[1]

Take a moment to think about every weight loss plan you have ever tried. Chances are that at one time or another, you were told to avoid something—fat, sugar, carbohydrates—and you listened.

You trimmed and skimped, curbed and cut back. Yet despite your dedication, you battled constant cravings. You endured fatigue, loss of energy, and poor health. And in the end, you managed to gain back every single pound you lost. Sound familiar? Now imagine a weight loss program designed to change all that.

Scientific research has proved that reducing the amount of calories we eat is the only way to lose weight and maintain our ideal body weight for life. But what we don't often hear is that nature has created an amazing nutrient that can help us do both of these things. It is called fiber.

By definition, fiber is the indigestible part of fruits, seeds, vegetables, whole grains, and other edible plants. But one could just as easily call it a miracle nutrient. Why? Because fiber and fiber-rich foods actually help regulate blood sugar, control hunger, and increase the feeling of fullness—all of which are essential to losing weight and keeping it off.

When I began writing *The Fiber35 Diet,* my goal was simple: to help as many people as possible achieve their weight loss goals using the power of this remarkable little nutrient. In fact, the Fiber35 Diet is based on eating 35 grams of fiber per day.

Although this sounds simple, you may be surprised to discover that the majority of Americans consume less than half that amount. Too many processed foods and refined sugars in our diet have taken the place of fiber-rich fruits and vegetables, leaving us vulnerable to weight gain and poor health. Don't beat yourself up, however, because you know you've been eating poorly and sugar has gotten a hold on you; the availability of processed foods and refined sugars is at record levels. It takes a conscious effort to seek out nutrient-rich super foods that will charge your metabolism and assist in your weight loss efforts. And I'm going to point you in the right direction by focusing on fiber, which will lead you down a path to superior health that goes beyond reaching your ideal weight.

By eating foods that collectively provide 35 grams of fiber per day, you will drop the weight you want to lose and maintain your ideal weight for the rest of your life. And by significantly boosting your daily fiber intake, you will reduce your chances of developing heart disease, stroke, high blood pressure, diabetes, cancer, and a host of other obesity-related conditions. I will have proved this to you by the end of the book.

The Fiber35 Diet begins with an eye-opening introduction to fiber and its role in weight loss. Then, I'll get right to the program and show you how you can start dropping pounds and gaining health with my Fiber35 Diet plan. You will learn a personalized weight loss equation—based on how many pounds you want to lose— that you will use to begin your journey toward eating healthfully and living well. I encourage you to consult with your physician prior to starting this program. It's helpful to have your doctor on board in your weight loss efforts; he or she can also provide additional support and advice tailored to your specific needs. You may, for example, have special health issues to consider and will need extra guidance from your personal health practitioner. I also encourage you to discuss your plans for starting an exercise program especially if you've been inactive lately.

This diet has three distinct phases—Phase One, Phase Two, and Phase Three. Each phase is discussed in detail, and I devote an entire chapter to the seven metabolic boosters, which are the ways you can enhance your results and optimize your fat-burning systems. Recommendations about supplements and nutritious food choices are included, as well as a variety of healthful and fiber-rich recipes for breakfast, lunch, and dinner. In addition, I have included a comprehensive strength and cardio training program designed to help you maintain your ideal body weight. By the time you arrive at Chapters 11 through 13, you'll be ready to go deeper into understanding just how this miracle nutrient is your helping hand in preventing disease and achieving vibrant health. You will be astonished by some of the research emerging to confirm the role of fiber in maintaining the body's machinery. Who knew that a zero-calorie ingredient could be so extraordinary?

It's true that in this country, and increasingly throughout the world, the number of people who are overweight or obese continues to grow at an alarming rate. And this is not just a health crisis; it's also an economic crisis that affects everyone, as the total costs attributable to obesity-related disease approach $100 billion annually.[2] But together, we can help stop this debilitating pandemic.

By beginning the Fiber35 Diet and adopting a lifetime eating system based on the remarkable health benefits of fiber, you are making a conscious choice: a choice to lose weight, to live better, and to take back control of your body. And I applaud that choice.

Your partner in optimum health,
Brenda Watson

Many of you may feel that it would take a miracle to lose weight and keep it off: and for you, I say fiber. Let me say it again. Fiber. Once more. Fiber. I can't say it enough, and here's why, plain and simple. Fiber is a powerful, natural substance that controls your hunger and eliminates calories *that you have already eaten*. Did you get that? Yes, fiber can actually "erase" calories you've already consumed and that could otherwise make you fat. The Fiber35 Diet returns you to the foods that Mother Nature intended you to eat in the first place. It's a plentiful diet, a delicious diet, and a diet so rich in nutrients that it helps you improve your health with every single bite, while giving you more energy than you have felt in years. In fact, if I could have another name for this book, it would be "The Energy Diet." Let's face it, who among us doesn't need more energy? I know you want to know the Fiber35 Diet secret, but first I want to tell you my story, and why it compelled me to write this book.

MY JOURNEY TO THE FIBER35 DIET

Twenty years ago, I was 25 pounds overweight, chronically tired, and suffering from health problems that would not go away. If the wind blew, I got a cold. If it rained, I couldn't sleep. When the seasons changed, my allergies were so bad I couldn't get out of bed. Forgive me for using a cliché, but I was sick and tired of being sick and tired. And so what I now consider the most important moment of my life (other than the birth of my two wonderful children and the day I met my husband) came on me one fall day when I was walking to the post office in Charlotte, North Carolina. Along the way, I decided to enter a new health food store that had opened in town, and it literally changed my life.

I remember that day as if it were yesterday. I made a decision that eventually resulted in my regaining control over my weight, my health, and my energy. Walking into that health food store was the first step in my personal journey to natural health, which twenty years later has seen me become an expert in natural nutrition by earning a degree in alternative health; found five natural health clinics; write four best-selling books on natural health; teach thousands of people across the world about the power of natural health, through hundreds of lectures and radio shows; and produce two national PBS television specials on the power of fiber and other nutrients for vibrant health.

What a wonderful journey it has been, and today, with the publishing of *The Fiber35 Diet,* I feel the most important chapter in my personal journey to share optimum health has been written. Why? Because, even after taking that initial step to improve my health and change my lifestyle, I again struggled with my weight. I felt as though I had gone to sleep at age forty-three and awakened at age forty-eight with an extra 30 pounds! Although, by then, I was well aware of the health benefits of fiber, it wasn't until this time in my life that I personally discovered the power of fiber in relation to weight loss. I began to incorporate more fiber, as outlined in this diet, and steadily the weight came off. Do I still struggle? All of you who have had to deal with weight problems know it takes a constant effort to maintain your ideal weight. I can honestly say the Fiber35 Diet has made that effort simple, effective, and rewarding.

THE SECRET TO A LIFETIME OF IDEAL WEIGHT

Today we suffer from an obesity epidemic that causes ourselves, our families, our communities, and our nation personal, emotional, physical, and even economic pain. We have become addicted to foods that first make us fat, then make us sick, and then kill us before our time. Enough is enough! The truth is that we all have the power to change our personal health destiny and you are starting right now!

For many years, through my natural health centers, I have been sharing the Fiber35 Diet Formula and have witnessed many people succeed. And you will succeed, too. Intuitively, we all know that food can be our medicine or our poison; and in my clinics, I have taught the simple truth about choice. We can all choose to eat ourselves into a state of obesity, fatigue, and compromised health, or to experience ideal weight, bountiful energy, and longevity.

Of all the things I have learned in the past twenty years, nothing is more powerful than the fact that optimum health begins and ends with what we eat and—of equal importance—what we do not eat. And of everything I have learned, the Fiber35 Diet is the most important information I could ever share with you. I applaud you for making a choice that I made twenty years ago: to take back control of your weight and your health, by learning information that will change your life, just as it did mine. What's the secret formula, exactly? Surely you've figured it out by now: 35 grams of fiber per day.

That's it! Simple and powerful. Wait until you see the results. This is the most powerful nutritional information I could ever share with you. The information is a magical seed that can grow into a life of improved health and weight. If I were on my deathbed, and a higher power said to me, "You can share one more message with the rest of the world. What will it be?" You guessed it: *Eat 35 grams of fiber a day!*

That's the secret. That's the diet. And here's how it works.

With the Fiber35 Diet, you are going to eat foods that collectively give you 35 grams of fiber per day. (To give you a basis for comparison, a raisin weighs about 1 gram.) In doing so, you can lose the weight you want to lose and then maintain your ideal weight for the rest of your life. And by eating a diet that provides you with 35 grams of fiber per day, you are going to reduce your risk of heart disease, diabetes, cancer, and a host of other obesity-related conditions.

Why will 35 grams of fiber a day be so powerful? There are two reasons:

1. **Fiber helps you restrict calories.**

2. **Fiber packs a miraculous one-two punch against disease.**

I'll be reiterating and exploring the science behind these two reasons throughout this book. Even though your immediate goal may be to lose weight, I want you to keep in mind that this diet will ultimately bring you long-term health.

Fiber and Calorie Restriction

It's a clinically proven fact that to lose weight, you must consume fewer calories than you burn. But you already knew this; it is conventional wisdom, and it has already been chiseled into your brain. The hard part is not knowing this fact but applying it to your life!

Your body is like a car: it gets a certain number of miles to the gallon. If you put more fuel into your tank than you need to drive, you will have extra fuel left over, which is stored in your body as fat. So when you want to lose weight, you must reduce your calories below the amount you need to fuel your body; and when you do, your body will tap your reserve tank (the weight around your middle, or your thighs, or your posterior) to obtain the fuel it needs to run. How do you do this? How do you reduce your calories? You eat 35 grams of fiber per day.

Of the many health miracles that fiber provides, appetite reduction may be the one you most appreciate, especially when it comes to losing weight. And it's not a drug or a synthetic medicine made in a laboratory for a pharmaceutical company. Fiber is Mother Nature's natural appetite reducer, and it's freely available. Fiber's powerful effects are going to allow you to comfortably reduce your calories in Phase One and Phase Two of the diet, where you will shed the pounds you don't want to carry around anymore.

The other essential element of this simple truth about weight loss is that you must burn more calories than you eat. If you restrict your calories but still don't burn more than you consume, you can't lose weight.

As much as we all would love to eat as much as we want and still lose weight, unfortunately our bodies are not designed that way. We require a certain number of calories to fuel our daily performance. Every activity we do burns calories. When we walk, talk, or even sit on a couch or sleep, we burn calories. When we think, we burn calories. In order for the heart to pump blood, we burn calories. All of our metabolic activities burn calories.

We gain weight when we consume more calories than we burn during any single day. We lose weight when we burn more calories than we consume. This fact is simple, and unavoidable. The larger the gap between the calories you eat and the calories you burn, the faster you will lose weight, and the more weight you will lose.

You already know this, too, and you also know that reducing calories during the period that you want to lose weight is just plain hard. Why is that? For one reason, when we reduce our calories below the number that we need each day to maintain our weight, a signal is sent from our brain that makes us hungry. The brain says, "Hey, where's all that food I need?" At the very time you have taken the steps to get rid of excess weight, your brain sends a starvation signal to make you that much hungrier.

From my experience, the difference between those who succeed and those who don't boils down to those who can control their appetite and those who cannot. If you could pop a pill that safely suppressed your appetite with no side effects (some drug companies have been trying to create such a drug for years), you'd want an endless supply of that pill, right? This is where the power of fiber begins. Fiber will help you to control your appetite in a natural way that is almost magical. It's as close to a magic pill as you're going to get, and it does a whole lot more than suppress your appetite.

Fiber as a Disease Fighter

Over the last forty years, food production actually increased faster than population.[1] And today, chronic and life-threatening diseases afflict millions of Americans. The statistics are breathtaking;[2] here's a glimpse:

More than 18 million have diabetes, which is the sixth leading cause of death in the United States. Millions more are prediabetic and don't even know it.

Almost 50 million suffer from chronic diseases like asthma or lupus.

About 70 million have arthritis, which is the leading cause of disability in the United States.

More than 80 million people in the United States suffer from digestive disorders like chronic heartburn, constipation, and irritable bowel syndrome, which happen to be the second leading cause of missed work (behind the common cold).

Here's an eye-opener: we spend more than $120 billion a year on medical care for digestive problems, and we spend nearly the same amount on fast food. What most people don't realize is that almost all of these digestive conditions result from inflammation of the digestive tract, an important topic I'll be covering. What does fiber have to do with this?

The value of a high-fiber diet came to the attention of the American public in the 1970s, when Dennis Burkett, MD, and his associates published their landmark research on the world's eating habits. Dr. Burkett noted that in indigenous cultures where dietary fiber intake is naturally high, people rarely suffered from obesity, heart disease, or colorectal tumors. Since then, studies clarifying the role of fiber in health and longevity have been pouring in and making sense out of all the anecdotal evidence. On the surface, fiber may not seem directly related to diseases like diabetes, asthma, and arthritis, and digestive disorders like heartburn, but there's a profound relationship between the state of your health and the quality of foods you choose to eat. Those high in fiber offer an array of disease-fighting benefits that can impact the chain of events that takes place in your body, which can possibly lead to any one of several chronic diseases that afflict millions of Americans.

If you want to prevent the big diseases that cut life short, fiber is your ally in two ways. First, each gram of fiber, by itself, has incredible health benefits, from helping to reduce your risk of cancer to cutting your risk of cardiovascular disease and diabetes. Second, fiber comes with an unbelievable bonus: it travels with disease-fighting friends everywhere it goes. When you go to the gas station, you have choices: regular, plus, or premium. The better the grade of fuel, the better your engine will run and the longer your car will last. Fiber-rich foods are the premium fuel in the nutrition world; quite simply, fiber-rich foods are the best fuel to power your body. Why is that? Because Mother Nature knows how to put food together; and where you find fiber, you find the energy-rich, disease-preventing nutrients that your body was designed to eat. And where you do *not* find fiber in food (other than beef, poultry, and fish), you usually find foods that make you tired, fat, and unhealthy. It's that simple, and that powerful.

We'll be going into greater detail about the impact of fiber on overall health a bit later on. I'll be taking you behind the scenes so you understand how, for example, fiber is associated with lower cholesterol, a better blood sugar balance, and enhanced immunity. For now I just want you to know that, as I've already noted, fiber packs a potent one-two punch.

It doesn't get any better than that!

Chapter 1 Summary

The Miracle Ingredient

- **Fiber's One-Two Punch**

  Fiber is the natural appetite suppressant that allows you to reduce calories; and reducing calories is the only way to lose weight.

  Fiber and its nutrient friends with whom it travels fight disease.

- **Fiber is a miracle in at least eight ways:**

  Fiber will help you lose weight.

  Fiber will help you maintain your ideal weight for life.

  Fiber reduces your risk of heart attack.

  Fiber helps maintain healthy cholesterol levels.

  Fiber reduces your risk of developing diabetes and helps maintain normal blood sugar.

  Fiber reduces your risk of cancer.

  Fiber promotes bowel regularity.

  Fiber helps improve your immunity.

- **The Fiber35 Diet Formula consists of eating 35 grams of fiber every day. This will help you lose weight and improve your health because:**

  Fiber controls hunger by acting as a natural appetite suppressant.

  Fiber eliminates calories we have already eaten.

  Fiber-rich foods are energy-rich, antioxidant-rich, disease-preventing foods.

CHAPTER 2

FIBER—THE AMAZING WEIGHT LOSS SOLUTION

When I first met Pete at one of my clinics, he weighed 210 pounds, stood six feet tall, and wanted to lose 30 pounds. As a restaurateur who constantly worked with food, Pete faced a daily challenge to keep his weight under control. He knew it was time to find a way of eating that would be satisfying and keep him fit for life. He impressed me because the first thing he said was, "What do I get to eat?" I liked that attitude, because when it comes to losing weight and managing weight for life, it's critical to focus on what you can eat, not what you can't. I asked Pete why he wanted to lose weight. He said to prevent heart disease. I loved that answer because as much as we all want to look good, in my experience, the people who maintain their weight loss are the ones who want it for health more than looks. At age forty-five, Pete was a father of two young children, ages nine and six, and he said it was important for him to have the energy to keep up with them. I also sensed that he wanted to make sure he'd be around to watch his kids grow into adults.

Because he wanted to lose the weight quickly, I put him on the Fiber35 diet right away and accelerated his weight loss by adding more exercise to his Phase One regimen. While following the plan and exercising every day but Sunday, he lost 3 pounds a week for six weeks, totaling 18 pounds. His weight loss continued in the next six weeks, and he dropped another 12 pounds—reaching his goal.

Two years later Pete reported back that he was maintaining his weight at around 190 and didn't feel deprived. My plan had changed his life. He said he was no longer afraid of being exposed to food all day long, because the issue wasn't willpower. The high-fiber foods he was eating satisfied him completely and eliminated the cravings that would otherwise lead to overeating. He even allowed himself to eat his favorite southern foods on Sundays, and he continued to eat six small meals daily. And if he ever veered off course for several days, as he admitted happened on occasion when he was traveling, he got right back on track and those extra pounds would go away. For me, hearing about his cholesterol level, which had dropped significantly with the diet and stayed that way, was the best news. Looks aside, having a body that is healthier and has been transformed, medically, is the ultimate reward for making a change in lifestyle. When friends and family members ask him how he does it, he's happy to share his secret.

WEIGHT LOSS MATH

Reducing your calories—i.e., going on a restricted-calorie diet—is the key to losing weight; there are no ifs, ands, or buts about it. Unless you reduce your intake below the number of calories that you need each day to maintain your current weight, weight loss is simply not possible (without a surgical procedure such as stomach stapling or liposuction). So the key to a successful weight loss program is to reduce your calories while you are trying to lose weight, and to eat no more than the calories that you need to maintain your weight once you have achieved your ideal weight. That's where fiber comes into play, because it helps you to reduce calories in four compelling ways:

1. **Fiber curbs your appetite, helping you to reduce intake.**

2. **Fiber actually helps reduce absorption of calories from the food you eat.**

3. **Fiber-rich foods are low-energy-density foods. In other words, you get to eat a lot of food without eating a lot of calories.**

4. **Fiber slows down your body's conversion of carbohydrate to sugar, thus supporting blood glucose stability to help you lose weight.**

That's quite a combination! Now you understand why I consider fiber a miracle ingredient when it comes to losing weight. Imagine—one ingredient halts hunger, reduces calorie intake from the food you eat, helps stabilize your blood glucose (and so reduces overeating), and allows you to eat plenty of food that is low in calories and high in nutrient-rich disease fighters. Let's take a look at each one of fiber's powerful weight loss factors in greater detail.

FACT: LEAN PEOPLE EAT MORE FIBER

The link between a lack of fiber in the diet and being overweight was obvious to Canadian researchers in 1995, when they conducted a clinical study at University Hospital in London, Ontario.[1] In this study, the researchers examined the fiber intake of three different weight groups: normal, moderately obese, and severely obese. Each group contained fifty people. The researchers kept detailed three-day food records that included everything each person ate, and then they analyzed how much fiber was contained in each day's food intake. Those in the normal group consumed significantly higher amounts of fiber—an average of 18.8 grams a day—whereas the moderately obese consumed 13.3 grams, and the severely obese 13.7 grams. The researchers concluded that dieticians and physicians need to emphasize the importance of a high-fiber diet to their obese patients.

THE CURB APPEAL OF FIBER

Cutting back on your calorie consumption is easier said than done. It's one thing to start reducing calories, but it's another thing to stay on the program long enough to achieve your goal and then maintain your new weight. Who among us hasn't experienced the yo-yo effect, losing, say, 10 pounds and then gaining them right back? Why is permanent weight loss so hard? Is it because of lack of motivation? Is it because of lack of willpower? Is it that you don't really want to lose weight? Of course not! The reason in most cases is what I call the *double-hunger-whammy*.

Double-Hunger-Whammy

The first hunger whammy happens when you decrease your caloric intake, particularly if you decrease it by a significant amount. Signals saying "Eat now" race through your body, and these signals can easily break down the willpower of even the most motivated and disciplined among us.

Actually, the sequence of events includes a few signals that dash through, ultimately creating a double whammy. The first signal races through the body's physiological express lane, screaming to the brain that it "needs more food." Your brain then responds by attempting to protect the body, sending out an "all points bulletin" that it's time to eat! These hunger pangs encourage you to do the very thing you're trying not to do—eat.

The "double" whammy in this is that your brain sends out another signal that's even more insidious, since you don't even know it's happening. Worried that it might not get the food it needs to keep you alive, your brain begins to operate in starvation mode and tells your body to slow down its metabolism, or the rate at which you naturally burn calories. So even though you are eating less, you begin burning fewer calories because your body is trying to conserve energy. It wants to hold on to food for as long as possible in case a famine ensues. The brain is one organ that can't go long without food, so it's not going to take any chances, and it's been programmed to react rapidly to signs of trouble—even if there really is no trouble. It will put out those fires burning in your metabolic engine quickly, leaving you operating in low gear and storing food as fat.

If you were actually unable to find food, this physiological double-hunger-whammy would be a life-protecting system and would help you survive the crisis; but when you are trying to lose weight in a world where calories are ubiquitous, it makes the challenge that much more difficult.

So let's talk about hunger. Other than thirst, there is no more powerful natural force on the planet than hunger. When you are restricting your calories to lose weight, eliminating hunger is the number one key to success. More specifically, the key is eliminating your hunger for food when your body doesn't need to be fed. And the Fiber35 Diet helps you to gain control of this balance between eating for nourishment and then stopping when your body has had enough. It's your weapon against the double-hunger-whammy.

Fiber: It's Hormonal

Physiologically, hormones control much of what you feel—moody, tired, hungry, hot, or cold. Women who are reading this know exactly what I'm talking about, and for that matter I am sure the men reading know it, too. Hormones are your body's messengers. They are produced in one part of the body, such as the thyroid, adrenal, or pituitary gland; pass into the bloodstream; and go to distant organs and tissues, where they act to modify structures and functions. Hormones act like traffic signs and signals—telling your body what to do and when, so that it can run smoothly and efficiently. Hormones are as much a part of your reproductive system as they are a part of your urinary, respiratory, cardiovascular, nervous, muscular, skeletal, immune, and digestive systems.

When it comes to hunger, there is a powerful hormone that helps regulate your satiety, the feeling of fullness that stops the hunger that causes you to eat. You know from experience that when you eat a lot of fiber, your hunger decreases. And most people believe this is because fiber occupies a lot of volume. So it's natural to think that its expansion in your stomach makes you feel full. But this is only part of the answer.

Fiber Turns On Your Antihunger Hormone

What most people don't know is that your small intestine produces a hormone that creates a feeling of fullness. It's cholecystokinin (kole-sisto-kinnen), abbreviated CCK. Think of cholecystokinin as a messenger that tells you, "OK, I'm full now, I'm not hungry anymore, so put down the fork." What a great messenger to have on your weight loss team. Well, as it turns out, fiber promotes and prolongs the elevation of CCK in the blood, and this elevation makes you feel full longer.

Cholecystokinin (CCK) is a gastrointestinal hormone that's responsible for stimulating the digestion of fat and protein. It is secreted by the first segment of your small intestine, the duodenum, which then causes the release of enzymes from the pancreas and bile from the gallbladder to aid in digestion. In fact, CCK mediates a number of physiological processes, and the good news about this hormone is that it suppresses hunger. It's what helps you push your chair away from the table without feeling deprived.

Among the first scientists to discover the effects of CCK was a team of researchers from the University of California, Davis. They found that women who ate a high-fiber meal released more cholecystokinin into their bloodstream than women who ate a low-fiber meal. The same was true of those who ate a high-fat meal as opposed to a low-fat meal. Have you ever noticed that when you eat a lot of fat, as in a big juicy steak, you feel satisfied? Well, fat releases the same hormone. Those who ate the high-fat and high-fiber meals reported a greater feeling of fullness, which was attributed to higher levels of CCK in their bodies.

This is pretty amazing, but you might be thinking, "What about men?" Same results. In another study, also conducted by the University of California, Davis, men were tested using a high-fiber meal and a low-fiber meal in a random order. Both the test meal and the control meal included eggs, bread, jelly, orange juice, milk, and margarine. The high-fiber meal contained white beans, whereas the low-fiber meal contained rice and dry milk. The researchers measured the subjects' levels of CCK before the meals and then for six hours afterward. Not surprisingly, the results indicated a CCK response that was twice as high after the high-fiber meal as after the low-fiber meal.[2]

Want more? Listen to this. Belgian researchers looked at one type of fiber in particular—oligofructose (OFS)—and discovered that it could help manage food intake in overweight and obese patients.[3] In their study, published in 2006, an equal number of men and women between the ages of twenty-one and thirty-nine were randomly assigned to a test group that got 16 grams of supplemental fiber a day for two weeks, or to a control group that got a placebo. First, the study found that during breakfast, fiber significantly increased the feeling of fullness among those who got the fiber versus those who got just the placebo. Second, the number of calories the test subjects ate at breakfast and lunch was significantly lower after fiber supplementation. And at dinner, the test group also reported higher feelings of fullness and reduced hunger. This meant they didn't eat as much, either. Not bad for just 16 grams of fiber supplementation per day!

Oligofructose is a subgroup of inulin, which is a type of fiber. Because it's on the more soluble side, relative to the general class of inulins, it's commonly used as an additive in yogurt and other dairy products.[4]

Other studies have confirmed these findings.[5] So the conclusion here is that you want to *increase* your levels of CCK as much as possible throughout the day so you can *decrease* your overall caloric intake and feel satisfied. And all this is possible, thanks to fiber. When you eat high-fiber foods, or a fiber supplement, you get the benefit of:

- **Increased volume in your stomach that makes you feel full.**

- **Higher levels of CCK that makes you feel full.**

Lowering your hunger levels is a key to controlling the calories you put in your body, which is exactly what fiber-rich foods help you do. This allows you to stay happily on a reduced-calorie diet long enough to reach your weight loss goal, and then to eat a normal amount of calories to maintain your weight in Phase Three, the Fiber35 Diet for Life.

THE FIBER FLUSH EFFECT

As powerful as fiber is in helping to control your appetite, it also has another special property, which sounds almost too good to be true. Fiber actually helps reduce absorption of calories from food that you have already consumed. Let me repeat that: fiber actually reduces calories you have already eaten! How can this be? Well, it seems that people who eat diets high in fiber excrete more calories in their stool. I know this is not a pleasant subject to discuss, but the technical term for this is *fecal energy excretion.* I call it the *fiber flush effect.* I first came across this in the early 1980s, in a book called *The F-Plan Diet,* written by Audrey Eyton. She found that the number of calories excreted from a high-fiber diet equaled 10 percent or more of the calories consumed during a given day.[6] The U.S. government has found the same effect, and other studies have also confirmed this phenomenon. The U.S. Department of Agriculture, for example, proved that consumption of 36 to 50 grams of fiber per day leaves 130 calories unused in the stool.[7]

Of all the studies done to show the "flush" effect of fiber on consumed calor the most thought-provoking one yet was by the Department of Human Nutrition and Food Science at the University of Kiel in Germany. There, researchers determined that for every gram of fiber you eat, you eliminate between 8.46 and 12.84 calories.[8] Mind you, the actual number of calories isn't exactly known; different studies have arrived at slightly different values. But when you do the math and take a conservative average of what various laboratories have calculated, it's reasonable to say that for every gram of fiber you consume, about 7 calories get eliminated in the stool.

To repeat: for every gram of fiber you eat, you can potentially eliminate 7 calories. This means that if you consume the 35 grams of fiber per day recommended in the Fiber35 Diet Plan, you could potentially eliminate 245 calories per day.

Now, let's take a look at what this means to you, using the average calculation that every gram of fiber will eliminate 7 calories per day from the total number of calories you have consumed. Over one month, if you eat at least 35 grams of fiber a day, you will eliminate 7,595 calories (245 calories x 31 days). Each pound of fat equals 3,500 calories, so every time you eat 3,500 *more* calories than you burn in any given period of time, you *gain* one pound; and every time you eat 3,500 *fewer* calories than you burn, you *lose* one pound. By eating 35 grams of fiber daily, you have the potential to eliminate 245 calories per day through your stool, which would add up to 7,595 calories in a month. That equals 2.17 pounds each month and 26.04 pounds per year. That's a lot of weight! Does it get any better than eating something that has no calories—fiber—and that actually subtracts calories from your body? I think not!

Seriously, How Does That Work?

You might be wondering how fiber manages to grab calories and rake them out of your body before they become a part of you. The mechanism is actually quite simple. What fiber is doing in this instance is blocking the absorption of calories consumed. Think of fiber as an escort that leads calories out of the body. Does this mean that fiber also grabs other things, like good nutrients and vitamins? Fortunately, there's been no evidence that fiber simultaneously prevents your body from retaining the nutrients it needs. In fact, the reverse has been shown: fiber can enhance your body's absorption of nutrients.

In 1985, British scientists examined how well iron, zinc, and calcium could get absorbed in a diet containing an extremely high-fiber mixture of bran, fruit, and nuts, which was recommended in Eyton's *F-Plan Diet*. They also looked at the absorption of the same minerals in a low-fiber diet. Not only did their study shoot down the idea that fiber could prevent the absorption of these particular minerals, but it also brought to light the possibility that fiber could increase the uptake of minerals in the diet. The absorption of iron and calcium in the high-fiber group was "significantly higher."[9] This may be due to the ability of fiber to slow digestion, actually allowing your body the time it needs to absorb minerals adequately.

BIGGEST BANG FOR YOUR CALORIE BUCK

Fiber-rich foods are the biggest bang for your calorie buck. Because fiber-rich foods are low-energy-density foods, they pack a high volume of content into a low-calorie package. In other words, you get to eat a lot of food without eating a lot of calories.

Different types of foods contain different amounts of calories. Technically, a calorie is the unit used to measure how much energy is produced when food is burned by the body. Think of your body as a machine that runs on the energy you put into it. I said earlier that the body is like a car, and it prefers premium gasoline. But you can give it too much energy for it to run efficiently, and then the excess energy gets stored for later use, in case you ever under-energize your body by taking in too few calories. As you can imagine, those unnecessary units of energy—calories—simply become fat. For those who really want to know what "energy density" means, here you go: energy density is "the number of kilojoules per unit weight of food, ranging from 0 to 37 kJ/g of food."[10] The rest of us can just consider energy density as the number of calories in a particular volume or weight of food. High-energy-density foods pack a lot of calories per bite; low-energy-density foods contain fewer calories per bite.

For example, a peach has fewer calories than a chocolate bar that weighs the same amount. Bite for bite, or ounce for ounce, you will gain more weight from eating ounces of chocolate than ounces of peach. Chocolate has a higher energy density than peaches. In fact, fiber foods are typically very low-energy-density foods (fewer calories per bite).

Energy Density

Three main food components determine energy density (ED):[11]

1. Water

2. Fat

3. Fiber

Most plant foods are high in water and fiber but low in fat and calories. They can make you full without making you fat. High-fat foods, which are usually low in fiber, are high-energy-density foods, with a lot of calories per bite. Both fat and fiber are very filling because they increase satiety and reduce hunger, but there is a marked difference in how they affect weight. Consider a crown of broccoli, which is high in fiber, versus a sticky bun of the same weight. They seem identical on the scale in terms of ounces, but they clearly are not the same on the calorie meter.

Because of the bulk that fiber adds to a meal, high-fiber (plant) foods generally have lower ED than high-fat foods. This is easy to understand when you consider that fat has 9 calories per gram, whereas fiber has *zero* calories! The critical fact in this concept of energy density is that "for a given weight or volume of food, fiber can displace the energy of other nutrients."[12] Therefore, a high-fiber meal that has the same weight as a low-fiber meal will make you feel fuller faster, and will provide you with fewer calories, while still giving you lots of nutrients. A bowl of steel-cut oatmeal with added flaxseed (high-fiber) will satisfy you more quickly than a bowl of white pasta that weighs the same. And ounce for ounce, the oatmeal will contain fewer calories than the pasta.

The Volumizer

You know intuitively that, generally speaking, feeling full is related to how much you eat, otherwise known as volume.[13] Think about it. If you were to eat a gallon of ice cream, you'd feel a lot fuller than if you'd eaten just a pint, right? The gallon has more volume. And because fiber increases volume without adding calories, you can lose weight without reducing the volume of food you normally consume, simply by substituting high-fiber foods for low-fiber foods. (Unfortunately, ice cream has little or no fiber, but you get the idea.) This is why the bowl of fiber-rich oatmeal would be lower in calories than the equivalent bowl of fiber-poor pasta. For the number of calories (roughly 270) that you get in a classic candy bar, you could eat almost 3½ cups of fresh blueberries.

This is important, because who among us does not like to eat? For most of us, the act of eating is one of the most enjoyable aspects of life. Who doesn't like sitting down in front of the TV and munching on a bag of potato chips? I know I do. The problem isn't necessarily the munching as such; it's the high energy density of the chips that ends up making us fat. So, why not munch on a bowl of cherries or raspberries? You get a delicious eating experience, without the experience of adding extra pounds.

Being able to eat, and eat a lot, is one of the keys to the Fiber35 Diet; and it is one of the reasons so many people have succeeded with a high-fiber diet when all other diets have failed. Eating is fun, and with the Fiber35 Diet you get to eat plenty!

Let's summarize again what we have learned so far:

- **Fiber curbs appetite, and suppressing your appetite helps you to reduce calories. Fiber does this by its sheer volume and its stimulation of the digestive hormone CCK, which promotes a feeling of fullness.**

- **Fiber actually eliminates calories from the food you eat, through fecal energy excretion (i.e., the fiber flush effect).**

- **Fiber foods are low-energy-density foods: they allow you to eat high volumes without high calories.**

- **And last but not least, fiber slows down your body's conversion of carbohydrate to sugar, and so it supports blood glucose stability and helps you lose weight.**

BLOOD CHEMISTRY STABILITY

The most notable hormone to gain attention in weight loss circles in recent years has been insulin. When you eat sugars and starchy carbohydrates (especially refined ones like white flour and table sugar), your body turns them into glucose (blood sugar) very rapidly. Glucose is the primary form of fuel for the body, and especially the brain. In response to the presence of glucose in the bloodstream, your pancreas secretes the hormone insulin, whose job is to unlock your tissues and escort glucose out of the blood into the tissue cells. Once glucose reaches the cellular level, any one of three things may happen:[14]

1. **It may be mobilized for immediate energy.**

2. **It may be converted to glycogen (stored sugar) for later use.**

3. **It may be stored as fat. This is the outcome you are probably most familiar with.**

Once your body's needs for immediate energy are met, excess glucose is converted into glycogen by your liver. This glycogen is actually stored blood sugar—glucose that is tucked away in your liver and muscles until your blood sugar level starts to drop. Once that happens, glycogen gets released from storage sites

into the bloodstream, providing glucose to bring blood sugar levels
glycogen storage sites are filled, your liver then converts any ren
to stored fat. This is the stuff of which the "spare tire" around th
made—and insulin is what facilitates fat storage.

If you overindulge in sugar or starchy carbohydrates at a me
level will rise sharply, but it will soon fall back. When this happ
experience a craving for more carbohydrates to bring your blood sugar back up
(offsetting the feelings of shakiness, fatigue, brain fog, and dizziness that go with
low blood sugar, or hypoglycemia). Habitual overconsumption of carbohydrates
sets off a repetitive pattern of quick rises and drops in blood sugar levels, which
causes your pancreas to work overtime releasing insulin.

As this pattern repeats itself over time, the effectiveness of insulin eventually
starts to decline. A condition of *insulin resistance* develops, in which your cells
become desensitized to insulin, making them ineffective at taking in glucose. The
net result is too much insulin in your blood. That insulin is unavailable for your cells,
however, because their insulin receptors have become blocked. With decreased
insulin sensitivity, adequate glucose is prevented from reaching your cells, and
so it cannot be used for energy. As a result, you feel tired. Your liver reacts to this
scenario by converting an increasing amount of glucose into stored fat. Before long,
you are tired *and* fat. The other bad news is that you are now at an increased risk
for high blood pressure, coronary artery disease, elevated triglycerides (blood fats),
low levels of "good" cholesterol, diabetes, stroke, breast cancer, polycystic ovarian
syndrome—and further weight gain.[15]

The good news is that fiber helps to slow down the conversion of carbohydrates,
so it can help reverse insulin resistance. High-fiber foods help normalize blood
glucose levels by slowing down the time it takes food to leave the stomach and
delaying the absorption of glucose from a meal. Fiber also increases insulin
sensitivity, which is the measure of how well cells respond to insulin and reduce
the level of glucose.[16]

Later on I'll go into greater detail about blood sugar balance, especially as it
relates to diabetes. Some of the research findings are astounding—proving how
powerful maintaining a healthy blood sugar balance can be in preventing diabetes
or even reversing its effects. And, as I will continue to show you, getting a healthy
dose of fiber can help achieve that balance.

Fiber—The Amazing Weight Loss Solution

- **Fiber curbs your appetite:**

    35 grams of fiber fights the "double-hunger-whammy."

    Fiber takes up a large volume in the stomach.

    Fiber promotes and prolongs cholecystokinin (CCK) to make you feel full longer.

- **Fiber eliminates calories you eat:**

    35 grams of fiber every day helps you eliminate calories that you eat.

    For every gram of fiber you eat, you can eliminate up to 7 calories.

    You can lose weight—perhaps as much as 26 pounds per year!—through what is called fecal energy excretion (fiber flush effect).

- **Fiber's low energy density makes you satiated by filling your stomach with lower-calorie foods. Fiber-rich foods contain more water, more volume, and fewer calories than potatoes, white rice, and other refined foods. That means you get to eat more food for less calories.**

- **Fiber slows down the conversion of carbohydrate to sugar. Fiber helps slow the conversion of carbohydrates into blood sugar, and this slowing allows glucose to be burned more efficiently instead of quickly being stored as fat.**

CHAPTER 3

WHAT IS FIBER?

Time to get up close and personal with fiber. If you had to define exactly what fiber is, what would you say? I'm talking about the dietary kind, which has nothing to do with muscle fibers or the fibers of a cotton shirt or spun glass.

The most basic definition I can give you is this: fiber is the part of food that cannot be digested or broken down into a form of energy for the body. This is why it has no calories. It is considered a type of complex carbohydrate, but it cannot be absorbed to produce energy. And it comes only from plants: fruits, vegetables, nuts, seeds, and grains. No animal products contain fiber. Specifically, fiber comes from a plant's cell walls. More technically, fiber falls into categories such as non-starch polysaccharides and several other plant components, including oligosaccharides, lignin, pectins, cellulose, waxes, chitins, beta-glucans, and inulin. But it isn't important you know these scientific names. We're going to focus on just two types of dietary fiber as they relate to the body—soluble and insoluble.

The fiber component of food is known as *dietary fiber.* Fiber is not technically a nutrient, since we cannot digest it. But while fiber itself contains no nutrients, the food in which it is found is loaded with them, and this is a powerful dietary connection. Where you find fiber, you find great health-giving nutrition. My goal with the Fiber35 Diet is to help you lose weight, but my number one objective is to share with you a diet that leads to lifelong health and everyday energy.

The fact is that where you find fiber, you find the world's most powerful health-giving nutrients, and with the Fiber35 Diet, you will nourish your body with more nutrients than you have probably ever had before.

FIBER TYPES AND SOURCES

There are two basic types of fiber—soluble and insoluble:

- **Soluble fiber (technically called pectin, gum, and mucilage) dissolves and breaks down in water. When this happens, it forms a thick gel.**

- **Insoluble fiber (technically called cellulose, hemicellulose, and lignin), also known as roughage, does not dissolve in water or break down in your digestive system. Insoluble fiber passes through the gastrointestinal tract almost intact.**

Remember: soluble fiber absorbs water, whereas insoluble fiber does not absorb water. Pretty simple.

Soluble Fiber

Functions of Soluble Fiber

Prolongs stomach emptying time so that sugar is released and absorbed more slowly

Binds with fatty acids, which are the building blocks of fats

Some Benefits of Soluble Fiber

Lowers total cholesterol and LDL cholesterol (bad cholesterol), thereby reducing the risk of heart disease

Regulates blood sugar

Some Food Sources of Soluble Fiber

Apples	Cranberries	Peaches
Barley	Lentils	Peas
Beets	Oat bran	
Carrots	Oranges	

Insoluble Fiber

Functions of Insoluble Fiber

Moves bulk through the intestines

Controls and balances the pH (degree of acidity or alkalinity) in the intestines

Some Benefits of Insoluble Fiber

Promotes regular bowel movements and prevents constipation

Removes toxic waste from the colon

Helps prevent colon cancer by keeping an optimal pH in intestines to prevent microbes from producing cancerous substances

Some Food Sources of Insoluble Fiber

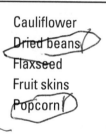

Cauliflower	Potato skins *(SWEE POTATOES)*	Whole grain cereals
Dried beans	Root vegetable skins	Whole grain oatmeal
Flaxseed	Sour plums	Whole grain pasta
Fruit skins	Wheat bran	
Popcorn	Whole grain breads	

You Need a Bit of Both

It's important to consume both soluble and insoluble fiber, because each type provides unique benefits, which we will discuss in more detail shortly. When you obtain the majority of your fiber through your diet, as you will in the last phase of the program, you will have a balance of soluble and insoluble fiber. This is what Mother Nature intended.

As I will explain in Chapter 10, if you supplement your fiber, look for a balanced fiber found in flax or a combination of flax, acacia, and oat fibers. I do not recommend psyllium because I have seen too many clients with too many complaints like gas, bloating, and constipation resulting from psyllium.

In Phase One and Phase Two of the Fiber35 Diet, you will use mostly soluble fiber in supplement form. In Phase Three (For Life), you will consume a balance of insoluble and soluble fiber.

Fiber works by two different mechanisms. Soluble fiber acts like a sponge, actually soaking up toxins as it passes through your gastrointestinal (GI) tract. Insoluble fiber does not break down in the digestive system; rather, it sweeps the GI tract, taking away toxins in the bowel as it encounters them. You can think of insoluble fiber as similar to a rake or broom—pushing toxins through. Insoluble fiber also tones the bowel by creating resistance, giving the muscles of the colon some exercise by providing something for them to push against. This increases the minute muscle contractions, also called peristalsis, necessary for good elimination. Hence, a blend of both soluble and insoluble dietary fiber makes for brilliant orchestration: collecting toxins and carrying them out when you have a bowel movement.

IS FIBER A LAXATIVE?

Most people think that fiber is a laxative, because many fiber products are advertised as aiding in the restoration of normal bowel regularity. The truth is that fiber is not a stimulant laxative; rather it is a type of carbohydrate that passes through your body undigested. In its transit through your gastrointestinal tract, it provides additional bulk, which gives the muscles of your GI system something to push against. It is this rolling or pushing motion, called peristalsis, that facilitates elimination through the colon. Many people ask, "With the Fiber35 Diet, will I go to the toilet all day long?" The answer is no. But most people find that they restore their elimination to one to three healthy bowel movements per day, which is best for optimum health.

Don't worry about counting grams of insoluble versus soluble fiber. You will never need to count fiber grams of each type, because by following the Fiber35 Diet as recommended, you will naturally get enough of each type during each phase.

Health Benefits of Soluble and Insoluble Fiber[1]

Soluble Fiber

Helps regulate blood sugar levels, lower cholesterol, and remove toxins.

Slows the absorption of food after meals and is therefore good for people with diabetes. It also removes unwanted metals and toxins, reduces the side effects of radiation therapy, helps lower cholesterol, and reduces the risk of heart disease and gallstones.

Insoluble Fiber

Helps prevent hemorrhoids, varicose veins, colitis, and constipation, and assists in the removal of cancer-causing substances from the colon wall.

Promotes weight loss, relieves constipation, helps prevent colon cancer, and controls carcinogens in the intestinal tract.

Helps lower cholesterol levels. It helps to prevent the formation of gallstones by binding with bile acids and removing cholesterol before stones can form, and it's beneficial for people with diabetes or colon cancer.

THE HISTORY OF HIGH-FIBER FOODS

There was a time when we naturally ate a high-fiber diet. This was when we ate from the farm, either our own or one nearby. But in the early 1900s, the processing and packaging of food became an enormous growth industry. Almost overnight, we went from eating fresh foods to eating processed foods. And almost overnight, our rates of obesity and diseases like heart disease, diabetes, and cancer skyrocketed. Today, processed food is the largest industry in the world, and is, unfortunately, an industry that processes a lot of fiber and other crucial nutrients out of our diet. Fortunately, you can make good decisions when it comes to rediscovering fiber in your food, and you don't have to give up delicious taste to do so.

SUGAR TRENDS

Between the 1950s and 1997, consumption of sugar and other caloric sweeteners rose 41 percent, to 200 pounds per person in 1997 in the United States.

Fruits and Vegetables

Put simply, there is no food group better for you than fruits and vegetables, and it's no coincidence that these food groups provide a lot of fiber. Earlier, I mentioned that fiber travels with disease-fighting friends. This is especially true of fiber-rich fruits and vegetables. The added bonus is that these foods are also rich in phytonutrients. By definition, a phytonutrient is simply any of the more than 1,000 nonnutritive chemicals produced by plants for their own protection. And phytonutrients help protect us, too. *Phyto* comes from the Greek word for plant. There are thousands of phytonutrients, and researchers are only now discovering what each one is and what their individual benefits are.

FRUIT AND VEGETABLE TRENDS
Americans increased fruit and vegetable consumption by 22 percent between the 1970s and 1997. There's plenty of wholesome produce to go around!

Phytonutrients at a Glance

As we will discuss later, phytonutrients are powerful disease-fighting compounds that are known to help prevent cancer and many other diseases. They are sometimes referred to as phytochemicals because biologically, you don't require them for survival. A lack of phytonutrients (unlike nutrients vital to human life) won't necessarily cause a deficiency disease, but phytonutrients are nonetheless essential to optimum health. These molecules have many and various health-giving functions in the body, playing important roles that keep it balanced and disease-free. For example, they may promote the healthy function of the immune system, act directly against bad bacteria and viruses, reduce inflammation, and be associated with the treatment or prevention of cardiovascular disease, among other ailments. In fact, some people believe that many of the diseases afflicting the populations of industrialized nations are due to a lack of phytonutrients in the diet. Part of the reason processed foods can be so unfriendly to our bodies and overall health is simply that naturally occurring phytonutrients have been stripped away during their manufacturing. The rise in treatable or preventable causes of death today—especially in western cultures where highly processed foods are abundant—may be related to phytochemical deficiencies in the diet.

Fruits and vegetables owe a lot of their vibrant colors to phytonutrients. Lutein, for example, makes corn yellow; lycopene makes tomatoes red; carotene makes carrots orange; and anthocyanin makes blueberries blue. The two ways in which phytonutrients help you is that they can (1) act as antioxidants and (2) reduce inflammation. Those that act as antioxidants offer protection from free radicals—the reactive, cell-damaging molecules that accumulate in the body and can lead to cancer. Indoles, a type of phytonutrient found in cabbage, stimulate enzymes that make estrogen less effective, possibly reducing the risk of breast cancer. Saponins, found in beans, interfere with the replication of cellular DNA, thereby preventing the multiplication of cancer cells. Capsaicin, found in hot peppers, helps protect DNA from carcinogens. And allicin from garlic has antibacterial properties.[2] These are just a few of the benefits phytonutrients can deliver.

The Dangers of Chronic Inflammation

Inflammation is a term we're hearing more and more these days, and it's been linked to weight gain and obesity. We're all familiar with the kind of inflammation that accompanies cuts and bruises on our skin—pain, swelling, and redness. If you suffer from allergies or arthritis you're also tuned in to what inflammation feels like. But inflammation goes much deeper than that and can happen in your organs and systems without your even knowing it—and without your really *feeling* it. And if you do feel it, it's in the form of an ailment or disease that you never thought started with general "inflammation."

Inflammation is supposed to be a good thing, as part of our body's natural defense mechanisms against foreign invaders such as bad bacteria, viruses, and toxins; but too much inflammation can be harmful. When inflammation runs rampant or goes awry it can disrupt your immune system and lead to chronic problems or disease. It may not seem remotely related to weight gain and obesity, but in fact, science is beginning to prove just how insidious chronic inflammation can be. Researchers are now discovering links between certain kinds of inflammation and the most pernicious degenerative diseases today, including heart disease, Alzheimer's disease, cancer, autoimmune diseases, diabetes, and an accelerated aging process in general. To put it simply, inflammation creates an imbalance in your body that stimulates negative effects on your health and your ability to lose weight.

A detailed discussion of inflammation is beyond the scope of this book, but I want you to keep in mind that what you choose to eat for nourishment is a factor in the level of inflammation your body experiences. Foods high in processed sugars and unhealthy fats, for example, can exacerbate inflammation. This, in turn, antagonizes weight loss and puts you at a higher risk for many other health problems. It also sets in motion a vicious circle that leads to more and more inflammation. The Fiber35 Diet points you toward the foods that will support the natural structure and functions of your body so that the body maintain a healthy balance, limiting inflammation and ushering in optimal wellness.

The Pennsylvania State University Department of Nutritional Sciences made the following statement about fiber-rich fruits and vegetables in relation to weight loss:

> *Given the recent surge in obesity, effective dietary strategies for weight management are required. Because fruits and vegetables are high in water and fiber, incorporating them in the diet can reduce energy density, promote satiety, and decrease energy intake.... Evidence suggests that coupling advice to increase intake of these foods with advice to decrease energy intake is a particularly effective strategy for weight management.*[3]

The message here is that eating high-fiber foods naturally delivers nutrients that contribute to your health. In this regard, perhaps the most powerful combination on the planet is fiber and phytonutrients.

In addition to fruits and vegetables, fiber is also found in whole grains and legumes (like beans). These are excellent sources of fiber, and they are part of the Fiber35 Diet to help you achieve 35 grams of fiber per day. Many people have an idea that it's difficult to consume 35 grams of fiber per day from food, but that is simply not true! The reason for this belief is that today we don't eat enough fruits, vegetables, whole grains, and legumes; instead, we eat too many processed foods that provide little if any fiber or nutrients. If you eat a regular bagel for breakfast, a hamburger and fries for lunch, and then pizza for dinner, your fiber tally for the day would be minimal.

High-fiber foods are also naturally low in fat. Fruits and vegetables are packed with an array of vitamins and minerals, especially vitamins A and C, the important B vitamin folic acid, and the mineral potassium. Whole grains are rich in vitamin E and the family of B vitamins. Legumes are naturally rich in iron and B vitamins, particularly B_6, as well as being a great source of protein and its many types of amino acids.

HOW MUCH FIBER DO WE NEED?

Here in the United States, our intake of fiber is typically quite low, about half of what it should be. The average American consumes an estimated 10 to 15 grams daily, whereas the amount recommended by the National Cancer Institute, the U.S. surgeon general's office, and many other professional health organizations is 20 to 35 grams per day. Can you consume too much fiber? Just how much is too much? No one knows for sure, but some authorities caution that amounts in excess of 50 to 60 grams may limit absorption of vitamins and minerals.[4]

I recommend a fiber intake of a minimum of 35 grams per day, which is higher than the low range of the generally recommended amount, but well below the level that some consider excessive. A diet with 50 to 60 grams of fiber should not be seen as unhealthy; it is generally beneficial and well tolerated by most people.

Water and Fiber Go Hand in Hand

One of the most common questions I hear when I recommend increasing fiber intake to 35 grams a day is, "Will I experience any side effects?"

When people experience gas, bloating, or constipation, the typical reason is insufficient water intake. For most people—those who drink enough water—increased intake of fiber relieves constipation. This is because fiber provides the bulk needed for peristalsis, the wavelike motion that moves food through your intestines. As you begin the Fiber35 Diet Plan, make sure you follow these guidelines:

- **Divide your body weight (in pounds) by two and drink that number of ounces of water per day. That means if you weigh 160 pounds, drink 80 ounces of water per day. You should do this even if you are not eating a high-fiber diet, but it is especially important when increasing your fiber intake.**

- **If you experience gas or bloating, take a digestive enzyme formulated specifically for gas and bloating, and increase your fiber intake more gradually.**

Add fiber slowly to reach 35 grams. If you become constipated, take a colon cleanse supplement before bed (cleanses will be explained in Chapter 9). You can also try a mineral-based laxative. Look for an all-natural laxative that contains minerals like magnesium (a stool softener) and gentle herbs like cape aloe and turkey rhubarb. It's really important to increase water intake as you slowly add in the fiber.

Now you know what fiber is and why it helps you lose weight. In Chapter 4, we will talk about how caloric restriction works, how much weight you are going to lose, and how fast you are going to lose it with the Fiber35 Diet.

Chapter 3 Summary

What Is Fiber?

- Dietary fiber is the indigestible parts of plant cells. Fiber is found only in plants, not in any animal products.

- There are two types of fiber: insoluble and soluble. Both are needed for health because they provide different benefits to the body.

- Supplementation with soluble fiber at the beginning of a weight loss program may improve your results.

- Foods containing fiber are rich in phytonutrients—chemicals made by plants that have antioxidant and disease-fighting properties.

- Many U.S. government agencies recommend consuming 20 to 35 grams of fiber every day.

CHAPTER 4

THE PHASES OF THE FIBER35 DIET PLAN

Over the past 20 years, most weight loss plans have asked you to count something. First it was grams of fat, then it was protein, and then carbohydrates. The bottom line is that to succeed at your weight loss program, the only clinically proven method is to restrict your calories. While it's important to eat the right kinds of fat, plenty of lean protein, and healthy carbs, at the end of the day whether you're going to tip the scales to the right or left depends on the number of total calories you've consumed. On the Fiber35 Diet, not only do calories count, but so do grams of fiber.

Counting grams of anything might sound like a lot of tedious math, but it's not. That's because I've made each phase of the Fiber35 Diet easy to follow by providing you with a variety of meal choices that have the right number of calories and grams of fiber. I have already done the counting for you, and a team of chefs made the food delicious by producing incredible recipes that you can use in any phase. So in truth, while the number of calories and grams of fiber are important to achieve, the counting has already been done. All you need is the desire to succeed!

To maintain their weight, most women must eat 1,500 to 2,000 calories per day, and most men must eat 2,000 to 2,500 calories. That is how much fuel is needed to keep up with your metabolism. If every pound of fat equals 3,500 calories, then if you want to lose one pound, you must eat 3,500 calories less than your body needs over a given period of time. For example, if you ate 1 calorie less than you need each day, it would take you 3,500 days (or 9.58 years) to lose 1 pound. But don't worry; with the Fiber35 Diet you can lose as much as 8 pounds a month.

Have you ever noticed that when you get a bad cold or the flu, you lose 3 to 5 pounds? That's because you eat less food than you normally would during the week or so that it takes for you to get better. If you need 2,000 calories per day to maintain your weight, then over a week (seven days), you would need 14,000 calories (7 × 2,000). When you're sick, you might eat only a bit of soup or some toast each day, and end up consuming a total of 500 calories, or 1,500 less than you need. Over a week, that's 10,500 fewer calories than your body needs to maintain your weight, and before you know it, you've lost 3 pounds (10,500 ÷ 3,500 = 3). Of course, no one wants to get sick to lose weight, but this is one way to understand the caloric math.

So I want you to keep this calculation in mind. For every 3,500 calories below your daily requirement that you restrict your intake, you'll lose one pound.

THE FIBER35 DIET WEIGHT LOSS GOAL FORMULA

In the Fiber35 Diet, there is something I call the *Fiber35 weight loss goal formula.* It's straightforward. You choose how many pounds you want to lose and multiply that number by 3,500; and this gives you the number of calories by which you will need to restrict your intake over a given period of time to lose your desired weight. Below, enter the number of pounds you want to lose on line 1. Then multiply that number by the 3,500 and enter the answer on line 2.

1. **Enter your weight loss goal in pounds:** _____

2. **Multiply your weight loss goal in pounds by 3,500:** _____

Do this now! That's right, get up off your chair, get a pen, calculate your goal, and write it in this book now. You have now begun your program. This is your magic number. I call it your *reduced calories goal,* or RCG.

THE FIBER35 DIET PHASES

The Fiber35 Diet has three phases. This gradual approach helps to insure that you will achieve your goal, and maintain it for life.

- **Phase One: Accelerated Weight Loss**

- **Phase Two: Moderate Weight Loss**

- **Phase Three: Lifetime Weight Maintenance**

Phase One of the Fiber35 Diet: Accelerated Weight Loss

In Phase One, you will reduce your calories by up to 1,000 a day. For example, consider an average man who needs 2,200 a day to maintain his weight. He will subtract 1,000 calories and consume 1,200 calories during this phase. This means that in Phase One, you will reduce up to 7,000 calories per week (seven days × 1,000 reduced calories per day). The result is that you will lose as much as 2 pounds per week (7,000 calories ÷ by 3,500 calories = 2). Please note that no matter what your starting point is, you should not go under 1,200 calories per day. For example, if you start with 2,000 calories you would reduce your caloric intake by only 800 calories a day in order not to go under 1,200 calories.

This is the most restrictive part of the program. In this phase, you will lose the most weight; and because you significantly cut down on your caloric intake, the pounds will drop off at the most accelerated rate. You don't think you can do this? Are you already picturing yourself chowing down at the refrigerator late at night? Don't panic. With the 35 grams of fiber that you will consume per day, you'll be able to control your hunger. In fact, you will be eating frequently; Phase One requires you to eat five to six times per day. And you will be staying in Phase One for up to one month. Most people will move into the second phase even though they will not yet have reached their weight loss goal. This program is designed to accelerate weight loss in Phase One, and keep the weight loss going in Phase Two. So once you complete a month in Phase One, you will move into Phase Two.

If you reach your target weight loss within the month of Phase One—hooray for you. You can either continue with Phase Two or go directly to the Fiber35 Diet for Life, Phase Three. Keep in mind that you do not have to spend the entire month in Phase One; however, I recommend that you spend a minimum of two weeks in this phase. If you prefer to move into Phase Two—eating a few more calories and achieving a more moderate weight loss—in the third or fourth week, you may do so.

Phase Two of the Fiber35 Diet: Moderate Weight Loss

In Phase Two, you will reduce your calories by up to 500 a day while still eating five to six times a day, and including your required 35 grams of daily fiber. For example, if you need 2,000 calories a day to maintain your weight, then you'll reduce that number by 500 calories to arrive at 1,500 calories per day in this phase. That means that in Phase Two you will reduce up to 3,500 calories per week (seven days × 500 reduced calories per day). You'll lose a little more than 1 pound a week, or approximately 4 to 5 pounds per month. Not bad! As in Phase One, do not go below 1,200 calories a day.

Phase Two has no definite end point. You can stay in this phase for as long as you need to reach your desired weight.

Want to lose even more? If you practice the Fiber35 Diet Metabolic Boosters during each phase, you can lose 1 extra pound every fourteen days, or about 2 extra pounds per month. I will go into detail about these boosters in Chapter 7.

Phase Three, the Fiber35 Diet for Life: Lifetime Maintenance

This is your new diet for life! You will not necessarily be reducing or counting calories, but you will continue to eat five or six times per day. By the time you reach this phase, you will have reached your weight loss goal. In the Fiber35 Diet for Life, you will maintain your ideal weight while continuing to eat a minimum of 35 grams of fiber per day.

PUTTING THE FIBER35 DIET PLAN TO WORK FOR YOU

Are you ready to put the numbers to work for you? To make sure that you thoroughly understand how easy the Fiber35 Diet plan is, let's repeat the Weight Loss Goal Formula.

Weight Loss Goal

Enter your Weight Loss Goal in Pounds (WLG).

Reduced Calories Goal

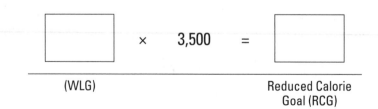

| | (WLG) | | Reduced Calorie Goal (RCG) |

Multiply the number of pounds you want to lose by 3,500.

This is your reduced calories goal, or RCG.

Number of Days to Achieve Your Weight Loss Goal

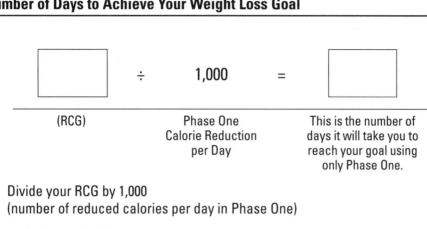

(RCG)	Phase One Calorie Reduction per Day	This is the number of days it will take you to reach your goal using only Phase One.

Divide your RCG by 1,000
(number of reduced calories per day in Phase One)

Example 1

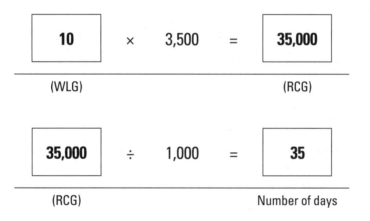

(WLG)	(RCG)

(RCG)	Number of days

Assume that you want to lose 10 pounds.

Multiply 10 × 3,500 calories (the number of calories in 1 pound of fat). The product is 35,000 calories. So the RCG is 35,000.

Divide 35,000 ÷ 1,000 (number of reduced calories per day in Phase One), to get 35.

That means it will take 35 days to lose 10 pounds using Phase One only.*

Example 2

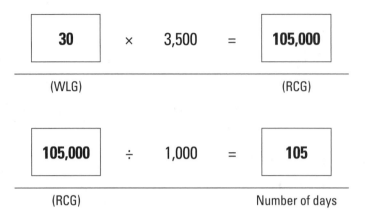

30 × 3,500 = **105,000**		
(WLG)		(RCG)

105,000 ÷ 1,000 = **105**		
(RCG)		Number of days

Assume that you want to lose 30 pounds.

Multiply 30 x 3,500 calories; the product is 105,000 calories, so RCG is 105,000.

Divide 105,000 ÷ 1,000 (number of reduced calories per day in Phase One), to get 105.

That means it will take 105 days (3.5 months) to lose 30 pounds using Phase One only.*

* In these two examples, I used Phase One to figure out how long it would take to lose 10 pounds or 30 pounds. But remember, the Fiber35 Diet is designed with three phases and each is very important. You will only stay in the first phase for up to one month—no matter how much you want to lose.

For most of my clients, I recommend all three phases. Of course, the first comment my clients have is, "I just want to do Phase One until I reach my goal." I understand this. Accelerated weight loss is attractive—the faster the better, right? But the way I look at it, with the Fiber35 Diet, you are going to lose every pound you want, and then maintain your ideal weight for the rest of your life, so what's the rush? I suggest that you stay in Phase One for no longer than one month. From the results I have seen over the years, using each phase of the program is always the best approach. There are two reasons why:

1. **Eating is fun, and you get to eat more in Phase Two than in Phase One.**

2. **Splitting your weight loss goal into Phase One and Phase Two helps stoke your metabolic fire, which in turn helps you lose weight in the short term and keep it off in the long term.**

Now that you have learned how the Fiber35 Diet Weight Loss Goal Formula works, let's learn more about calories, metabolism, and how to calculate exactly how many calories you need each day to maintain your weight.

WHAT ARE CALORIES?

The word *calorie* has long been intimately associated with dieting. Before counting grams of fat, carbohydrates, and protein, dieters counted calories. This was and still is the only way to lose weight. So let's take a look at exactly what a calorie is and how it's related to body weight.

As I already noted in an earlier chapter, calories are the way we measure the energy value of our food. Quite simply, we could not survive without the calories we obtain from food. Technically, a calorie is the amount of energy, or heat, required to raise the temperature of 1 gram of water by 1 degree Celsius (or 1.8 degrees Fahrenheit). Think of a calorie as a unit of energy. When we think of a cheeseburger as "600 calories," that is a measure of the potential energy it contains. A burger contains each of the three types of macronutrients: protein, fat, and carbohydrates. Each type of macronutrient contains a specific number of calories.

Carbohydrates	Protein	Fat
1 gram = 4 calories	1 gram = 4 calories	1 gram = 9 calories

All foods are made up of one or more of these three macronutrients, which are essential nutrients the body needs in relatively large quantities. If you are cooking at home and know the macronutrient composition of the foods in your meal, you can calculate the number of calories by adding together the calories present in the total number of fats, carbohydrates, and proteins. But who has time for that? In this book you'll find ample recipes for everyday living. If you use the recipes, you will not have to count anything—no calories, and no grams of fiber for that matter. Calories and fiber are provided for each recipe. And if you want to use your own recipes, I have provided visual calorie and fiber counters in charts for 100 different foods that allow you to calculate fiber grams and calories just by looking at your recipe. Use the daily journal template in Appendix A to write down your tallies as you plan your meals and snacks.

Many Food Options, but Only Three Building Blocks of Life

Our eyes look at food in different ways, but our bodies look at food in only one way. While we see a steak, a pizza, and a Caesar salad as different foods, our bodies see each as just an amalgam of energy in the form of protein, fat, and carbohydrates. Once we eat, our bodies go to work breaking down our meals into smaller units of energy that are transported into the bloodstream to provide the fuel we need to operate. From the time we begin chewing, digestive enzymes are secreted to break our food down into its component parts:

- **Carbohydrates break down into glucose and other simple sugar molecules.**

- **Fats break down into glycerol and fatty acid molecules.**

- **Proteins break down into amino acid molecules.**

Once this breakdown occurs, the resulting molecules are transported to the cells via the bloodstream. Either these molecules will be absorbed by the cells for immediate use, or they will be stored as fat.

CALCULATING YOUR CALORIC REQUIREMENTS

When we discuss how many calories we need per day, we're actually talking about how many calories our cells need to function as they should. Although everyone's caloric needs are slightly different from everyone else's, food manufacturers base the nutritional information on their labels (otherwise known as percent daily values, or %DV) on a 2,000-calorie diet, which represents the caloric needs of the "average" person.

What makes a person "average"? Well, for a woman, average is defined as someone who needs to eat about 2,000 calories a day to maintain her weight, whereas an average man is defined as needing approximately 2,500 calories. In the years I have worked with clients to help them lose weight, I have found this number to be roughly accurate; however, there are several factors that determine the exact number for each individual.

So while I'm going to explain the technical way to determine your personal daily caloric requirement (to maintain your weight), it will not influence how to put the Fiber35 Diet to work for you. Whether or not you know your exact caloric requirement, you can still follow the eating program in Phase One and Phase Two as described. Those who do want to know their exact number should read on. (For those who don't, it's OK to move on to Chapter 5.)

There are several things that influence how many calories you need per day to maintain your weight:

- **Height**

- **Weight**

- **Gender**

- **Age**

- **Activity level**

The mathematical formula that helps you determine your personal daily caloric needs takes into account most of the factors listed above, and is calculated using two variables: your metabolic rate (MR), and the amount of energy expended during physical activity.

Your MR, which accounts for about 60 to 70 percent of your body's daily energy expenditure (calories burned), is the rate at which your body uses energy to maintain basic life processes like heartbeat, normal body temperature, and respiration. The formulas used for calculating MR are different for women and men because men have more lean muscle mass than women. In general, if you're a woman, your metabolism burns 10 calories per day for every pound of body weight; if you're a man, your metabolism burns 11 calories per day for every pound.[1] This means that a woman who weighs 150 pounds would burn 1,500 calories (150 × 10) just to run her body's core functions, and a man of the same weight would burn 1,650 (150 × 11). This is one reason why men find it easier to lose weight—they naturally burn more calories, even when they are inactive.

The second variable for calculating caloric needs—energy expended during physical activity—would ideally take into account all physical activities in which a person engages, even seemingly insignificant ones like fishing and playing the piano. To get an idea of your daily caloric needs, take these three easy steps.[2]

Step 1: Calculate Your Metabolic Rate (expressed as "resting calories," or RMR)

For Women

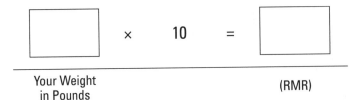

Your Weight in Pounds   (RMR)

Multiply your weight in pounds × 10 = RMR
(A 140-pound woman would have an RMR of 140 × 10, or 1,400.)

For Men

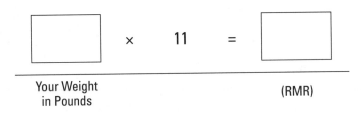

Your Weight in Pounds   (RMR)

Multiply your weight in pounds × 11 = RMR
(A 140-pound man would have an RMR of 140 × 11, or 1,540.)

Step 2: Calculate Energy Expenditure During Physical Activity (expressed as "activity calories")

How much energy do you use up during the day in various activities? To figure this out, determine if you are sedentary, somewhat active, or moderately active.

- **Sedentary: You barely get out of a chair during the day.**

- **Somewhat active: You engage in activities such as walking around frequently during the day, light gardening, playing with children, light swimming, etc.**

- **Moderately active: You engage in activities such as brisk walking several times a week, light exercise, sports activities, heavy yard work, swimming laps, etc.**

Multiply your MR number (from step 1) by the percentage attached to the description below that fits you best, as follows.

Sedentary

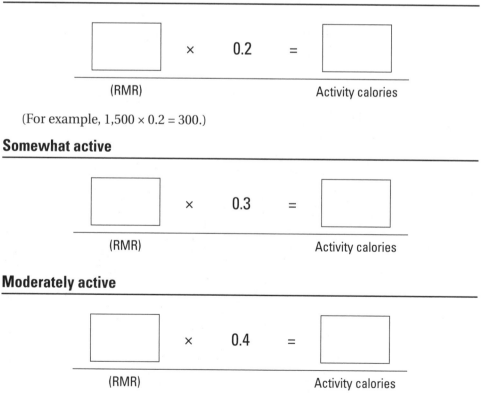

| | × | 0.2 | = | |
| (RMR) | | | | Activity calories |

(For example, 1,500 × 0.2 = 300.)

Somewhat active

| | × | 0.3 | = | |
| (RMR) | | | | Activity calories |

Moderately active

| | × | 0.4 | = | |
| (RMR) | | | | Activity calories |

Step 3: Add Up the Results of Steps 1 and 2

Add the results of step 1 and step 2 to arrive at the total number of calories you potentially burn in a day to maintain your current weight.

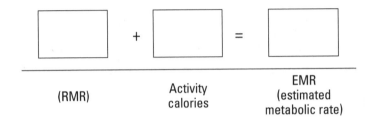

| | (RMR) | | Activity
calories | | EMR
(estimated
metabolic rate) |

For example, a 175-pound inactive woman would have an EMR of 2,100:

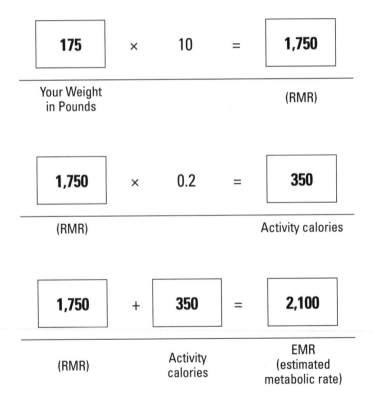

Now, with this information in hand, you're almost ready to start the Fiber35 Diet! But first, we must learn about the Fiber35 optimum nutrition food choices.

Metabolism is the sum of all the biochemical processes of an organism. Our bodies are incredibly complex in their functioning. Most of the functions that keep us alive are microscopic in nature, but all of them require energy, which we measure as calories. The first controlled experiments in human metabolism were published by Santorio Santorio, an Italian physician, in 1614 in his book *De statica medicina,* bringing him fame throughout Europe.

Chapter 4 Summary

The Phases of the Fiber35 Diet Plan

- **Every pound of fat equals 3,500 calories.**

- **To lose weight you must reduce your calories.**

- **The Fiber35 Diet has three phases:**

    Phase One, accelerated weight loss. During this phase, you will reduce up to 1,000 calories per day. You stay in this phase for up to one month.

    Phase Two, moderate weight loss. During this phase, you will reduce up to 500 calories per day. You remain here for as long as it takes to reach your goal weight.

    Phase Three, weight maintenance. During this phase, you will maintain your weight by consuming 35 grams of fiber every day. This is your plan for life!

- **Calories are energy values in food. Fiber does not contain any calories.**

- **You can use simple calculations to determine not only how much weight you will lose in each phase, but also how much time you will take to lose it!**

CHAPTER 5

THE FIBER35 DIET OPTIMUM NUTRITION FOOD CHOICES

When Joy started the Fiber35 Diet, she was twenty-seven years old and weighed 140 pounds, which was about 14 pounds more than the ideal weight for her height and frame. She expected to be hungry all the time on my plan because that's how she had felt on every other diet she'd tried. But she was pleasantly surprised, and the plan soon became a lifestyle that was easy to maintain. After just two weeks on the program she reported feeling better than she had felt in years, and said her energy level rivaled that of her two Jack Russell terriers. Dropping 2 pounds a week, she got down to a healthy weight of 126 pounds in seven weeks and never felt as if she was "on a diet." She says, "When I first started the Fiber35 Diet, I expected to be hungry all the time but that wasn't the case. It satisfied my hunger and never left me feeling 'stuffed,' which was actually quite nice. And I didn't fall back into my old poor eating habits." Ten months later, Joy remained at her ideal weight. Her energy level continued to soar, making her fifty-hour workweek much easier and more enjoyable.

Ultimately, the key to maintaining your ideal weight for life is to eat plenty of the right foods and few of the wrong foods. As Joy learned, finding a system of eating that's satisfying and easy to maintain is the secret to a lifetime of good eating. In this chapter, I summarize the principles of the Fiber35 Diet for Life and give you the core knowledge to make the right food choices for you and your family. If you turn to Chapter 14, you'll see that I have provided many recipes; also, you can get new recipes every month online at www.fiber35diet.com. You could simply use these recipes and enjoy optimum nutrition, but I encourage you to learn the principles behind them, which are presented here. These food choices should keep you lean and healthy throughout your lifetime.

Some of the foods listed in this chapter will be restricted in Phase One and Phase Two of the diet. In Chapter 6, you'll get the details of the restrictions for each phase. For now, we're simply concerned with healthy food choices.

PROTEINS + FATS + CARBS + FIBER

The Optimum Nutrition Food Choices are simple. You primarily eat:

1. **Lean protein**

2. **Fats:**
   healthy oils
   nuts and seeds
   dairy (moderate consumption)

3. **Carbohydrates/35 grams of fiber for life:**
   fruits
   vegetables
   legumes/beans
   grains (consume with caution)
   fiber supplements

When you follow the above Optimum Nutrition Food Choices, your daily diet will consist of approximately:

- **25 percent protein. Two or three servings (3–4 ounces per serving) of poultry, fish, and red meat (use sparingly).**

- **25 percent fat. Two or three servings of seeds and/or nuts, totaling 1 ounce daily, good oils (1–3 tablespoons daily); ¼ avocado; lean proteins (as described below).**

- **50 percent complex carbohydrates. Six to eight servings of fruits, vegetables, legumes; two or three servings of whole grains (½ cup = one serving).**

Protein

Protein is crucial for good health. Your body uses protein for every process it undertakes. Twenty percent of its structure is protein-based. Literally every body part—including blood, enzymes, muscle, skin, organs, and antibodies, as well as hair and fingernails—requires protein, so you need to make sure you get plenty in your diet. The key again is to get protein from good sources.

Meats and fish are the richest sources of protein. In general, a serving of these foods should be about the size of a deck of cards. Experts agree that you should eat two or three servings of protein-rich foods every day. Each serving should be 3 to 4 ounces of cooked meat.

Get your protein from lean sources like fish and poultry. Stay away from fatty meats. These include red meat and cheese, which should be eaten infrequently. For most Americans, protein makes up about 10 percent to 15 percent of daily calories. I recommend that 25 percent of your calories come from protein-rich foods, especially if you are following the Fiber35 Diet Strength Training Program. Athletes trying to build large amounts of muscle may need even more.

When I began to regain weight as I aged, I had to adjust the size of my meat portions. I found that even though I was eating high-quality meats, I was eating too much.

Protein Construction

Proteins can be relatively large, convoluted molecules. But their basic building blocks are natural compounds called amino acids. The proteins used by the human body require twenty amino acids. The body can make eleven of these amino acids; the remaining nine, known as essential amino acids, have to come from food.

Meat and other animal foods are said to contain complete protein: this means that they contain all of the essential amino acids. Individual vegetarian foods are technically incomplete because they are missing at least one essential amino acid.

As a rule, although meats contain a complete protein, they are not necessarily better for you than the protein found in vegetarian foods. Many types of meat are high in saturated fat, and all are completely devoid of fiber. Foods from plants are usually rich in fiber and contain vitamins and antioxidant nutrients that meat lacks.

In the past, nutrition experts have recommended that vegetarians carefully combine different types of foods to ensure that they eat complete proteins. More recently, researchers have come to believe that as long as you eat a wide variety of fruits, vegetables, beans, nuts, and seeds, you are assured of getting all the necessary amino acids. You can get an adequate supply of protein if you don't eat meat; if you avoid fish as well, then you simply have to focus on other sources of quality protein, such as eggs, whey protein, and legumes. Meat lovers typically don't have a problem getting their protein; but it's not that difficult for vegetarians to get their protein, especially with today's access to a multitude of nutritious food options.

Acceptable Sources of Protein	Protein Foods to Avoid
Chicken	Fatty cuts of meat
Beef—use sparingly	Honey-baked ham
Eggs	Liver
Fish—especially salmon	Processed lunch meats
Pork—use sparingly	
Tofu—use sparingly	
Turkey	
Whey	

I recommend wild salmon instead of farm-raised salmon, as the latter contains excessive amounts of arachadonic acid and omega-6 oils, both of which can be linked to increased levels of inflammation. We already get too much omega-6 in our diets as it is. You must ask your grocer if the salmon is wild.

Go for Grass-Fed

When you eat red meat, your health will benefit more if you choose meat from grass-fed rather than grain-fed animals. Since the introduction of factory farming, large cattle-raising operations have mainly fed grain to their livestock because it's cheaper and makes animals fatter and heavier. That practice means more profits for food companies. Consequently, most of the cuts of meat in supermarkets are from grain-fed animals.

However, the meat from grass-fed animals is more nutritious than the meat from grain-fed animals. It contains more conjugated linoleic acid (a component of fat that boosts fat burning and the buildup of lean muscle mass), more omega-3 fats, and vitamin A. In addition, it has less fat, cholesterol, and calories. Farms that specialize in grass-fed cattle are also better for the environment. Cattle allowed to graze on large areas of land are easier on the land and pollute less than do factory farm animals.

In choosing chicken and other poultry, you'll want to look for the meat (and eggs) of grass-fed rather than grain-fed animals; you'll also want to be certain that the animals are free-range, meaning that they roam freely in the outside environment, rather than being cooped up in factory farms, in overcrowded and often inhumane conditions. (See Appendix C, Resource Directory, for sources of meat, poultry, and eggs.)

What Protein Portions and Serving Sizes Should Look Like

While we recommend two to three servings of protein daily, men and women have slightly different protein needs. Therefore, recommendations regarding their serving sizes differ somewhat, as indicated below:

Serving Sizes

	Beef:	Chicken/poultry:	Fish:
Women	2 ½ ounces	2 ½ ounces	2 ½ ounces
Men	3 ½ ounces	3 ½ ounces	3 ½ ounces

Note: Eggs are a recommended source of protein. There is no need for restriction of eggs unless your doctor orders it. We have delicious egg white recipes in the recipe section, and you can have whole eggs as you stabilize your weight.

When you are eating protein-rich foods, you want to always combine them with fiber-rich vegetables—since meat, you will recall, has no fiber. As your weight becomes more stable, you can begin to add starchy vegetables, such as sweet potatoes, or whole grain bread if you desire. However, you'll want to continue to stay away from refined white sugar and white flour products.

Fats

Let's clear something up: dietary fat is *not* an impediment to losing weight. Eating the wrong kinds of fat, and too much fat, is what leads to weight gain. Just as there are good and bad carbohydrates, there are also good and bad fats. And just as the low-carb diet fad biased us against all carbs, the low-fat diet fad has negatively influenced our general view of fats.

Fat has received more than its share of negative publicity during the past few decades. As Americans keep gaining weight, volumes have been written about the evils of fat. But for your good health, you need to understand the truth about this misunderstood nutrient. Not all fats are created equal, so let me give you some guidelines.

Avoid Trans Fats (Hydrogenated Oils)

Some fats are quite harmful. Not surprisingly, researchers have found that the least desirable types of fats are man-made. These are the trans fats, also known as hydrogenated fats. Manufactured from polyunsaturated fats (which are good fats), they have been chemically altered by food companies so that they stay solid at room temperature (think of margarine). They are added to cookies, doughnuts, and other processed foods, and are used to make desserts more moist and crackers more palatable. Hydrogenated fat also lengthens the shelf life of processed baked foods like pastries, cookies, and crackers, which can sit longer in stores before turning rancid. Many commercially prepared fried foods like chips, french fries, and onion rings may also contain large amounts of trans fat.

Studies show conclusively that trans fats raise your risk of both heart disease and cancer. Many studies have found that eating trans fats causes a rise in blood fats immediately following consumption, increasing the risk of heart problems, and that trans fatty acids also causes a drop in HDL—the good cholesterol that can help protect the heart and arteries.[1]

The negative effects of trans fats have finally begun to be formally acknowledged by governments around the world. Denmark has actually outlawed trans fats. Canada is working on a similar ban. The United States now requires that food labels list the amount of trans fats, and soon the United States may outlaw these fats.

EFFECTS OF TRANS FATS ON THE LIVER

Researchers believe that what goes on in the liver to produce cholesterol and triglycerides—two types of fat—is stimulated by the consumption of trans fat. In addition, researchers at the Harvard School of Public Health found that people who ate the most trans fats also had the most inflammation in their bodies, as well as constricted blood vessels.[2] Both of these factors can increase your chances of developing heart disease.

Limit Saturated Fats

Saturated fats are those found in red meats and dairy products like milk, eggs, cheese, and butter. A telltale sign of saturated fats is that they remain solid at room temperature. Most researchers believe you should limit the total amount of saturated fat in your diet, and I certainly agree. Eating saturated fat boosts the overall level of cholesterol, which—as you're aware by now—is associated with an increased risk of cardiovascular disease.[3]

On the other hand, the effect of saturated fat on your health may also depend on the foods you generally consume with it. Researchers at Stanford University showed that eating the typical American diet while merely trying to limit saturated fat was not as effective as adding an abundance of fiber-rich vegetarian foods.[4] In other words, a high-fiber diet offsets some of the negative effects of saturated fat.

I'm not going to ask you to cut out foods with saturated fat, like red meat and cheese, completely. You just need to cut back on how much of this fat you eat. If you want to have your cheddar cheese and a juicy steak, limit your portions according to guidelines given, and make sure you eat plenty of fiber-rich vegetables at the same time or take a fiber supplement along with your meal.

Enjoy Good Fats

Unsaturated fats are the good fats—fats that you should make sure to include in your diet every day. There are two kinds of unsaturated fats: polyunsaturated and monounsaturated.

Polyunsaturated fats are liquid at room temperature, and their use lowers the total amount of cholesterol (both LDL and HDL). The best sources of polyunsaturated fats are flax oil, pumpkin seeds, oily fish, walnuts, and hemp oil. These oils also contain omega-3 fatty acids. Other sources of polyunsaturated fats include soy, corn oil, safflower oil, and sunflower seeds. Consuming foods with polyunsaturated fats, especially oily fish, has been shown to lower inflammation and actually benefit people with disorders related to inflammation.[5]

Remember: although inflammation is a survival mechanism our bodies use to prevent infection from foreign invaders like bad bacteria, viruses, and toxins, it tends to spin out of control in the context of our modern lifestyles. A poor diet and a sedentary lifestyle, for example, can cause chronic inflammation in the deepest corners of our bodies where we don't detect the inflammation until it's diagnosed later on as heart disease, dementia, diabetes, obesity, or one of any number of degenerative problems that can derive from inflammation. Chronic inflammation can displace the natural state of our immune system and create an imbalance in our bodies that in turn can lead to a variety of health problems. Science is just beginning to tell us how dangerous inflammation can be when it goes unchecked. Anything that can help us lower our levels of inflammation and perhaps prevent further inflammation in the future is a good thing.

Monounsaturated fats, like polyunsaturated fats, are liquid at room temperature. They are excellent for cooking because they can withstand heat, whereas some polyunsaturated oils (like flaxseed oil) are heat-sensitive. The best sources of monounsaturated fats are olive oil, canola oil, and peanut oil. Olive oil is your best choice for all-around use. Monounsaturated fats lower bad cholesterol (LDL) and raise good cholesterol (HDL), reducing the risk of heart disease. They also can lower the risk of diabetes and other chronic illnesses.

Minimizing intake of your saturated fat (from meat) and eating more monounsaturated oil (like olive oil) and polyunsaturated fats (like fish and flax oils) lowers the risk factors for a number of chronic illnesses, helps you maintain a healthy weight, and provides a more balanced intake of omega-3 and omega-6 fatty acids.[6]

Fish oil—composed of polyunsaturated fats known as omega-3s—has long been recognized as one of the most important sources of healthy fats. In fact, a large study found that people with heart disease who took a gram of fish oil in a supplement daily for several years decreased their risk of a fatal heart attack by 25 percent.[7]

Americans eat about 110 pounds of meat per capita annually, twice as much as Europeans.

Fish Oil and Health

As far back as anyone can remember, the Norsemen of Scotland, Greenland, and Scandinavia took spoonfuls of cod liver oil to stay healthy during the brutally cold winters. The descendants of those Norsemen brought this custom with them when they settled along the Atlantic coast of North America. Like their ancestors, they knew that a spoonful of cod liver oil has multiple benefits.

As scientists now recognize, cod liver oil, along with fish oil, contains the omega-3 fatty acids eicosapentaenoic acid (EPA) and docosahexanoic acid (DHA). Cold-water marine animals like mackerel, salmon, cod, flounder, albacore tuna, sardines, and anchovies are rich sources of omega-3s. These fatty acids are also found in seaweed and microalgae.

Another type of omega-3, alpha linolenic acid (ALA), originates in vegetarian sources including flaxseed oil, chia seeds, and dark green leafy vegetables like kale and turnip greens. Studies indicate that the body can usually convert the ALA found in plants to EPA. However, some people do lack the enzymes (desaturase and elongase) needed for this conversion. Fish oils are a better choice than other sources of omega-3s, as they don't require conversion.

TAKE OMEGA-3 TO BURN STORED OMEGA-6 FATS

The best way to burn away fat stored in your body is by displacing it with the good fats from fish or fish oil supplements. In other words, new fat helps clear out "old" fat—especially the kind hiding in peripheral tissues around the belly, thighs, and bottom—a fascinating recent discovery by researchers at Washington University School of Medicine in St. Louis.[8] The increase in omega-3 can help your body eliminate excess stored omega-6s more efficiently, and also reduce harmful inflammation.

The body uses both EPA and DHA as building blocks for prostaglandins, hormonelike substances that regulate the dilation of blood vessels, inflammation, and other critical processes. By reducing inflammation, EPA and DHA help reduce the risk of heart disease, the pain and swelling of arthritis, and the risk of some types of cancers. DHA is also essential for normal brain development in babies.

Americans in general don't consume nearly enough omega-3 fats; the overwhelming majority of our diet contains omega-6s. Omega-6 fats are found primarily in vegetable oils and grains. When you consume too much omega-6 in foods like corn oil, your body may release chemicals that promote inflammation. (An exception is gamma linolenic acid from borage oil, which can lower inflammation.)

A large number of experts believe that many of our health problems are linked to the omega-6 fats in our diet. Our intake of omega-6 has doubled in the last six decades, while consumption of omega-3 has dropped. This lopsided situation may partly explain the drastic increase in chronic illnesses in the past fifty years. Dietary reliance on omega-6 foods has been linked to high blood pressure, water retention, depression, and increased blood clotting.[9]

The lesson here is that you should eat plenty of fish, or take a fish oil supplement, to get your omega-3s. If you take a fish oil supplement, make sure it contains the enzyme lipase to help digest the oil. It should also be enteric-coated if possible. By that I mean it's coated with a material which allows it to pass through the stomach without getting destroyed by the stomach acids, and enter the small intestine where it gets released. Also, eat heartily of foods containing unsaturated fats that are necessary for good health (see the chart below).

CUT OUT THE BAD FATS, AND GET PLENTY OF GOOD FATS

Cutting out all fats without regard to quality doesn't lower the risk of heart disease. In the Women's Health Initiative Trial, about 50,000 postmenopausal overweight women between the ages of fifty and seventy-nine were studied for eight years. The researchers found that reduced total dietary fat did not decrease the risk of heart disease, stroke, or coronary vascular disease.[10] The study did find a reduction in heart disease in women with reduced intake of saturated and trans fats or higher intake of fruits and vegetables.

Fat Sources: The Good, the Bad, and the Ugly
(Serving Size = 1 to 3 tablespoons per day)

The transition to good oils is a very easy one. Use your flax oil as a salad dressing; use olive oil for cooking; and take fish oil supplements, 2 grams per day, for added benefit.

Oils to Use Regularly	Oils to Use Sparingly	Oils & Foods to Avoid
Olive oil*	Soy oil	Any hydrogenated oil
Canola oil	Butter	Chips
Flax oil*	Coconut oil	Fried foods
Peanut oil	Corn oil	Margarine
	Cottonseed oil	Processed foods
		Shortening

Do not cook with flax oil—use it on salads and foods after cooking. Cook with olive oil at low heat.

Note: Flax and olive oil are highly recommended. Try to use canola oil rather than corn oil when you can. (See Resource Directory for preferred sources of healthy oils.)

Coconut Oil Is a Surprisingly Good Fat

Don't be afraid to use coconut oil once in a while. For a long time it was wrongly associated with many of the "bad" saturated fats, and was unfairly accused of being a potential cause of increased cholesterol levels and increased risk for heart disease. But the opposite is actually true, as it's been shown to *lower* cholesterol and support a healthy heart.

Coconut oil has been consumed in the tropics for thousands of years. It was once prevalent in western countries, including the United States; popular cookbooks advertised it at the end of the nineteenth century. With a long shelf life and a melting point of 76 degrees Fahrenheit, it was a favorite in the baking industry. But a negative campaign against saturated fats in general—and the tropical oils in particular—led most food manufacturers to abandon coconut oil in favor of the polyunsaturated oils that come from the main cash crops in the United States, particularly soy.

The attitude toward coconut has shifted now that studies prove just how beneficial this oil can be. Studies of native diets show that indigenous populations are generally in good health, and don't suffer from many of the modern diseases that plague western nations. In fact, people who live in tropical climates and have a diet high in coconut oil have less heart disease, cancer, and colon disorders.

Current studies of this oil show that it can have anticancer, antimicrobial, and antiviral effects.[11] It may reduce cholesterol and stimulate your thyroid to support your efforts at weight loss. The secret to coconut oil's germ-fighting characteristics is lauric acid, the most prevalent fatty acid found in the oil. Lauric acid is also prominent in the saturated fat of human breast milk, giving vital immune-building properties during a child's first stage of life. Except for human breast milk, nature's most abundant source of lauric acid is coconut oil.

In the 1940s farmers tried using coconut oil to fatten their animals but discovered that it made the animals lean and active and increased their appetite. Oops! The farmers then tried an antithyroid drug, which made the livestock fat with less food but was found to be a cancer-causing agent. By the late 1940s, farmers noticed that the same antithyroid effect could be achieved by simply feeding animals soybeans and corn.

Nuts, Seeds, and Avocados

Nuts, seeds, and avocados are all excellent sources of healthy oils, but because of their high fat content, you'll want to consume them in moderation, following the portion guidelines given in this section.

Select raw, natural, or organic nuts and seeds (like pumpkin, sesame, and sunflower) whenever possible, and soak them overnight to deactivate enzyme inhibitors and thus improve their digestibility.

To Be Eaten Regularly

Avocado	Raw almond butter	Raw macadamia nuts
Mixed nuts and/or seeds	Raw almonds	
Peanut butter	Raw hazelnuts	

Nut butters and nuts are in the same category, so choose one or the other. Do not eat both on the same day.

Nut, Nut Butter, and Avocado Portions and Serving Sizes

Food	Serving	Size
avocado	¼	
nuts/seeds	1 ounce	12 walnuts or 24 almonds
nut butters	1 teaspoon	1 thumb tip
nut butters	1 tablespoon	3 thumb tips

FAT AND OIL TRENDS

The average use of added fats and oils in 1997 was 47 percent above what it had been in the 1950s.

Dairy

Dairy products fall into the categories of both protein and fats. Although full-fat dairy products are more nutritious than reduced-fat versions, they're not conducive to weight loss. So you're going to want to choose no-fat or low-fat dairy products while you're on this diet. We always recommend organic dairy. If you are using full-fat dairy, use it sparingly, as a condiment—for example, sprinkle Parmesan cheese on a dish.

Some people do not digest dairy products well; they lack an enzyme needed to break down the lactose found in milk products. As a result, they experience a lot of gas and bloating when they eat dairy. If you choose to eat dairy, and you are one of these people, you may benefit by taking a natural lactose digesting enzyme when you consume the dairy. We recommend substituting almond or rice milk for cow's milk, especially if you are lactose-intolerant.

In recent years, the dairy industry in the United States has been heavily advertising milk as beneficial to weight loss. Some research, however, disputes this claim.[12] Preferred dairy products include the following:

What Dairy Portions and Serving Sizes Should Look Like

Food	Serving	Size
Cottage cheese	½ cup	½ baseball
Hard cheeses	1½ to 2 ounces	6–8 dice
Kefir	1 cup	1 baseball
Parmesan cheese	3 to 4 tablespoons	1½ to 2 whole walnuts
Ricotta cheese	¼ cup	1 golf ball
Soy milk	1 cup	1 baseball
Plain yogurt (unsweetened)	One 8-ounce container	

The above amounts may need to be reduced in Phase One of the diet.

Carbohydrates/35 Grams of Fiber

The proportion of carbohydrates in the program (50 percent) might be surprising to you, given the low-carb brainwashing that has unfortunately occurred in America. The key is to get the right carbs, rather than limit carbs. The right carbs, those considered complex, are exactly the foods that you need to prevent disease and get your 35 grams of fiber per day. Fruits and vegetables are Mother Nature's natural medicines. Earlier, we talked about the benefits of fiber in managing and maintaining our weight. Without carbohydrates in your diet, it would be nearly impossible to get adequate fiber. Let's briefly review the four basic ways in which fiber can help you lose weight and keep it off:

1. **Fiber controls your appetite through the hormone CCK.**

2. **Fiber removes calories with your bowel movement. We call this the fiber flush effect.**

3. **Fibrous foods are energy-dense.**

4. **Fiber helps regulate blood sugar.**

There are five ways in which we will take in fiber daily:

1. **Fruits**
2. **Vegetables**
3. **Beans**
4. **Grains**
5. **Fiber supplements**

Fruits

Fruits are high in fiber and water. They are also loaded with disease-fighting phytonutrients. Following is a chart of the fiber content of commonly consumed fruits.

Fiber Content of Fruits
(Serving Size = 1 medium piece of fruit or 1 cup of fruit)

You'll want to consume two or three servings of fruit daily. A good idea for a snack is to combine yogurt or nut butter with fruit. See our snack ideas in the recipe section.

As you can see from the chart below, some fruits have much higher fiber content than others. This is something you need to understand, so that you can make good choices.

Fruit	Size or amount by volume	Total fiber
5 to 10 grams of fiber		
Coconut	¼ cup	10 grams
Orange	1 medium	7 grams
Grapefruit	½ large	6 grams
Raisins*	½ cup	6 grams
Dates*	½ cup	6 grams
Kiwi	2 medium	5.2 grams
Apple	1 medium	5 grams
Blackberries	½ cup	5 grams
Persimmons	1 medium	5 grams
Elderberries	½ cup	5 grams
Honeydew melon	½ melon	5 grams

Fruit	Size or amount by volume	Total fiber
2.5 to 4 grams of fiber		
Banana	1 medium	4 grams
Papaya	½ large	4 grams
Pear	1 medium	4 grams
Raspberries	½ cup	4 grams
Cantaloupe	1 medium	4 grams
Carambola (star fruit)	1 medium	3.5 grams
Currants	½ cup	3 grams
Tangerine	1 medium	3 grams
Apricot	3 medium	2.5 grams
0 to 2 grams of fiber		
Blueberries	½ cup	2 grams
Cranberries	½ cup	2 grams
Mango	1 medium	2 grams
Nectarine	1 medium	2 grams
Peach	1 medium	2 grams
Plum	2 medium	2 grams
Strawberries	½ cup	2 grams
Tomato	1 medium	2 grams
Cherries	½ cup	1.5 grams
Pineapple	½ cup	1 gram
Grapes	½ cup	< 1 gram

* These are high-glycemic-index foods, and therefore should be eaten sparingly. By definition, a high-glycemic food is broken down into simple sugar and moved into the bloodstream quickly. This process typically involves a surge of insulin, which rushes out from the pancreas to take care of the high-glycemic carbohydrate.

Vegetables

Limit starchy vegetables. These are higher in calories—and higher in glycemic index, which means that they get absorbed into the bloodstream rapidly and cause a surge in insulin. They also tend to be lower in phytonutrients. Starchy vegetables include potatoes, sweet potatoes, corn, and winter squash. They contain about 140 calories per cup.

The chart below gives the fiber value of many vegetables. Select according to your preference, and eat liberally from a wide variety of high-fiber vegetables, emphasizing non-starchy vegetables.

Fiber Values of Vegetables
(Serving Size = 1 cup raw vegetables or ½ cup cooked vegetables)

You may eat freely of all non-starchy vegetables, but you will need to be moderate with starchy ones if they are consumed alone. Try to eat four to six half-cup servings per day of vegetables.

Vegetable	Size or amount by volume	Total fiber
2 to 5 grams of fiber		
Acorn squash*	½ cup, cooked	4.5 grams
Sauerkraut	½ cup	4 grams
Sweet potato*	1 medium	3.5 grams
Potato*	1 medium	3 grams
Corn*	½ cup, off cob	3 grams
Beets	1 medium	2.5 grams
Broccoli	½ cup	2 grams
Brussels sprouts	½ cup	2 grams
Carrots*	½ cup	2 grams
Cauliflower	½ cup	2 grams
Eggplant	½ cup	2 grams
Rutabaga	½ cup	2 grams
Spinach	½ cup	2 grams
Turnip greens	½ cup	2 grams

Vegetable	Size or amount by volume	Total fiber
Less than 2 grams of fiber		
Collard greens	½ cup	1.5 grams
Yellow squash	½ cup	1.5 grams
Mustard greens	½ cup	1.5 grams
Cabbage	½ cup	1 gram
Celery	½ cup	1 gram
Kale	½ cup	1 gram
Leek	½ cup	1 gram
Popcorn*	1 cup, popped	1 gram
Zucchini	½ cup	1 gram
Lettuce	½ cup	0.5 gram
All precut packaged lettuce mixes	½ cup	0.5 gram

These starchy vegetables have a high glycemic index. Therefore, you'll want to use them sparingly, especially if eaten alone. Eating these starchy vegetables with other foods, especially fats and protein, will substantially lower their glycemic index.

Beans/Legumes

Legumes, like grains, contain substances called phytates, which are considered anti-nutrients. Phytates bind to, and therefore block the absorption of, vitamins and minerals like iron, magnesium, vitamin B, and calcium. To counteract this so that you can take advantage of the high fiber legumes offer, soak them overnight. Soaking will remove most of the phytates.

Fiber in Legumes
(Serving Size = ½ cup)

Serving sizes of beans are very important, as they are high in calories. Whe
eating beans, limit your servings to ½ cup.

Legumes (beans)	Amount by volume	Total fiber
Red bean	½ cup	9 grams
Adzuki	½ cup	8.5 grams
Lentil	½ cup	8 grams
Crowder peas	½ cup	8 grams
Mung	½ cup	7.7 grams
Black	½ cup	7.5 grams
Pinto	½ cup	7.3 grams
Chili	½ cup	7 grams
Garbanzo (chickpeas)	½ cup	7 grams
Great northern	½ cup	7 grams
Kidney	½ cup	7 grams
Lima	½ cup	7 grams
Navy	½ cup	6 grams
Anasazi	½ cup	4.5 grams
Appaloosa	½ cup	4.5 grams
Field peas	½ cup	4 grams
Green peas	½ cup	4 grams
Edamame (soy)	½ cup	3.8 grams
Green bean	½ cup	2 grams

A Note about the Glycemic Index

When it comes to carbohydrates, the term *glycemic index* often arises. What does this mean? The glycemic index measures how fast carbohydrates are broken down into simple sugars and moved into the bloodstream. Foods with the highest glycemic index are simple sugars and processed grain products like regular pasta and white rice. These foods cause a rapid rise in blood sugar after a meal; they may also cause a hormonal change that stimulates hunger and leads to overeating. The surge of insulin alone can trigger intense food cravings and make it very difficult to control your eating.

That said, the concept of the glycemic index isn't as exact as you might think. For example, a regular bagel would be considered a high-glycemic food. But when it is topped with lox or a spread of almond butter, the entire chemistry of the meal can change, resulting in a food that's lower on the glycemic index. Hence, glycemic index ratings are accurate only when no combining of foods takes place, and so the system is a bit unpractical. That's why we're not going to worry too much about the glycemic index. It's not a reliable dietary guide, and it can become confusing. In fact, the American Diabetes Association does not recognize the glycemic index as an educational tool in the treatment of diabetes. That says a lot.

AVOID ARTIFICIAL SUGARS
Try to avoid artificial sweeteners. Even though they contain zero calories, they have hidden side effects. Popular artificial sweeteners like aspartame can cause rashes, headaches, and stomach cramps, and change bowel function. What's more, artificial sweeteners have also been known to increase appetite and mess with brain chemistry. Although scientists continue to debate this topic, one study at Purdue suggested that artificial sweeteners can actually impair your body's natural ability to "count" calories on the basis of a food's sweetness, so it's harder to judge how many calories a certain food has, and thus harder to adjust intake accordingly.[13]

Grains

Grains, like dairy products, are allergens for a number of people. Many grains, which include breads, cereals, and pastas, contain gluten. Gluten intolerance is one of the most common and underreported allergies in the United States. But its discovery has given rise to the production of a number of gluten-free foods, which is good news for people bothered by gluten.

GRAIN AND FLOUR TRENDS
Consumption of flour and grain products increased from 155 pounds per person annually in 1950 to 200 pounds per person annually in 1997 in the United States.

The other problem with grain-based foods is that the vast majority of them are made with refined flours. This means that the beneficial fiber has been removed during processing, significantly increasing the food's score on the glycemic index. Foods like this set off the sugar-insulin-fat storage cascade that affects most overweight people. If you choose to eat grains like pasta, cereal, or bread, make sure that they are made with whole grains, preferably sprouted whole grains, and keep the use of these within your daily caloric requirement.

As has been discussed, when it comes to grains, you want to limit yourself to whole-grain options, totally avoiding products made with white flour. Remember to soak your grains overnight before cooking them the next morning, as you would do with beans, to deactivate phytates. Also, soaking makes the grains cook very quickly in the morning. I choose steel-cut oatmeal in the morning, and the cooking time is only five minutes after soaking overnight.

Fiber in Grains *(Serving Size = ½ cup)*

You'll want to consume two or three servings of whole grains per day. I highly recommend non-gluten grains for anyone sensitive to gluten. There are a number of tasty, nutritious, high-fiber whole grains from which to choose, as indicated in the chart below.

Grain, dry	Amount by volume	Total fiber
Amaranth	½ cup	17.2 grams
Barley	½ cup	12 grams
Teff	½ cup	16 grams
Spelt	½ cup	16 grams
Rye	½ cup	12 grams
Wheat bran	½ cup	12 grams
Oats	½ cup	12 grams
Millet	½ cup	10 grams
Bulgur	½ cup	8 grams
Quinoa	½ cup	6 grams
Brown rice	½ cup	4 grams

In addition to the above sources of fiber, cold cereals can be a super way to start the day with a fiber-packed meal. (Refer to Resource Directory for the best choices in fiber-rich breakfast cereals.)

Fiber Supplements

It's important to strive for 35 grams of fiber daily in your diet not only to achieve a healthy weight, but to prevent disease. Today, everyone is in a hurry, and we don't always obtain the full 35 grams from our diets. This results in a need for fiber supplements to make up the deficit. Here are your major choices:

- **Fiber wafers**
- **Sprinkle fiber**
- **Bars**
- **Shakes**

The first two options consist of soluble fiber, conveniently packaged for people who are away from home a lot. The bars and shakes are snacks and meal replacements with high fiber content. With these choices available, no one should fall short of achieving the desired daily intake of 35 grams of fiber.

In Chapter 10, I'll cover these supplements plus others in more depth. It's easy to obtain these supplements at most health food stores and incorporate them into your daily regimen.

SAMPLE DAILY FIBER INTAKE OPTIONS

Now that you know where to find fiber, let me show you how easy it to get 35 grams per day from your meals. Below is a sample of high-fiber foods that could be included in one day of delicious eating. (Because you will avoid starchy vegetables like winter squash during Phase One, this is more typical of what you could eat during Phase Two or on the Fiber35 for Life.)

High-Fiber Foods

Food	Portion	Fiber
Oats	3 ounces	9 grams
Orange	1 medium	7 grams
Apple	1 medium	5 grams
Acorn squash	½ cup, cooked	4.5 grams
Banana	1 medium	4 grams
Broccoli	1 cup	4 grams
Red beans	¼ cup	4 grams
	Total fiber	37.5 grams

In this example, you have a bowl of oatmeal and a banana for breakfast. You have an apple for a snack and then a lunch that includes a chicken breast topped with provolone cheese plus some curry squash. You eat an orange as a snack and then have a lean steak for dinner with broccoli, plus a salad with red beans and ranch dressing. Not a bad day of eating, and presto—37.5 grams of fiber!

Let's look at another example.

More High-Fiber Foods

Food	Portion	Fiber
Apple	1 large	7 grams
Orange	1 medium	7 grams
Corn	1 ear	5 grams
Raspberries	½ cup	4 grams
Sweet potato	1 medium	3.5 grams
Whole grain toast	1 slice	3 grams
Kiwi	1 medium	2.7 grams
Beets	½ cup	2.5 grams
Blueberries	½ cup	2 grams
Broccoli	½ cup	2 grams
Lettuce	2 cups	2 grams
Spinach	½ cup	2 grams
Cabbage	½ cup	1 gram
Total fiber		43.7 grams

In this day of bountiful eating while in the Fiber35 for Life phase, you wake up to a breakfast of a cheese omelet, turkey bacon, whole grain toast, and fruit salad. You have an apple as a snack, and then for lunch you have a big delicious rainbow salad with chicken. It's okay that you've exceeded the 35 grams of fiber on this day. As I noted earlier, you'd have to eat in excess of 50 to 60 grams of fiber for it to be considered excessive. And it would be quite a challenge to consume that much in a day! It's far easier to consume too little than too much, and I'd rather see you eating a bit more than 35 grams a day than a tad below. Consider 35 as your minimum; if you can get in 40 to 45, that would be a bonus. However, I do not generally reccomend going over 60 grams of fiber. You'll have an orange as a snack, and for dinner a turkey burger with baked sweet potato fries and corn on the cob. The result: a delicious day of eating and 43.7 grams of fiber. Amazing!

The meal plans and recipes in this book have this all figured out for you, but suffice it to say that 35 grams of fiber a day is a delicious and nutritious way to eat.

Fiber and Calories

Once you get started on this plan, you'll automatically become a whiz at reading nutrition labels and distinguishing between the good and the not-so-good. Be careful about eating foods that are high in calories but are disguised as "healthy" because the package says something like "good source of fiber." The rule of thumb here is to seek foods that have at least 2 grams of fiber per 100 calories. Following is a chart to guide you.

Fiber and Calories

If an amount of food contains:	And the fiber amount is:	The grade is:
100 calories	4+ gram	Best
	3 grams	Better
	2 grams	Good
	1 gram	Bad

Watch your sodium intake: the RDA is 2,400 milligrams a day! Read labels even when a package says "low sodium."

WARNING: SUGAR AND SOFT DRINKS

Sodas can pack a ferocious punch of calories. The a 64-ounce "Big Gulp" soft drink sold at convenience stores can account for as much as 900 or 1,000 calories in just one serving. It's possible to consume more calories from soda and other sweet drinks than from any other food. And diet drinks, while they are a better alternative than regular sodas, are not necessarily a safe bet. Artificial sugars commonly used in diet sodas can trigger a sugar craving and lead to blood sugar imbalances. Studies have also shown that the risk of becoming overweight increases by a whopping 41 percent with each can of diet soda consumed daily.[14]

While you're on the Fiber35 Diet, it's hugely important to severely limit undesirable high-carbohydrate processed foods. These include white bread; white rice; pasta that is not whole grain; refined breakfast cereals; sugary desserts; crackers; and any foods, like sodas and candy, that contain concentrated sugar and corn syrup. These products, which are based on white sugar and white flour, not only prevent you from losing weight but also rob you of your health. This is because their natural fiber content and many important nutrients have been removed during the refining process. The result in the body is an inability to properly metabolize carbohydrates, creating toxic conditions and making it difficult to lose weight.

Alcohol has the same disrupting effect as refined carbohydrates on blood sugar. Once you've achieved your weight loss goals, however, you may well be able to tolerate moderate consumption of sugar and alcohol. Only you can determine if you are among those who can tolerate these items in moderation.

Dark chocolate and red wine (a glass a day) have been shown in studies to confer certain health benefits, so their use in moderation, particularly on special occasions, should not be harmful. And, in fact, dark chocolate does provide some fiber. Try to eat chocolate with a high percentage of cocoa. A serving of strong dark chocolate (70 percent cocoa) has 4 grams of fiber.

Identify and eliminate foods to which you are or may be allergic or sensitive. These can contribute to weight gain and cause health problems.

In Chapter 15, you'll find a comprehensive shopping list that you can take to a grocery store or another market. In that chapter, you'll also find weekly menu plans for guidance through each phase.

PORTION TRENDS[15]

Obviously, since we Americans are taking in more calories from more food, our portion sizes have increased. (So too have plate sizes!) Consequently, today's typical serving sizes are vastly different from those of the 1950s, as the data below indicate:

Food	1950s	Today
Average fast-food burger	1 ounce	6 ounces
Average soda	8 ounces	32–64 ounces
Average theatre serving of popcorn	3 cups	16 cups
Average muffin	less than 1 ounce	5–8 ounces

The fast-food burger of today contains approximately 546 calories. A side of medium fries has about 413 calories. If we add a soda to our order, another 154 calories are consumed, for a total calorie count of over 1,100. This is more than half of the daily calorie requirement for many people, especially those who are inactive.

Chapter 5 Summary

The Fiber35 Diet Optimum Nutrition Food Choices

- **By eating according to the Fiber35 Diet Optimum Nutrition Food Choices, you will be avoiding processed foods, limiting consumption of meats, seeking high-quality foods, and reaping the benefits of 35 grams of fiber.**

- **The Optimum Nutrition Food Choices include:**

    Lean protein

    Fats

    - healthy oils
    - nuts and seeds
    - dairy (moderate consumption)

    Carbohydrates/35 grams of fiber for life

    - fruits
    - vegetables
    - legumes/beans
    - grains (consume with caution)
    - fiber supplements

CHAPTER 6

GETTING STARTED WITH THE FIBER35 DIET

Congratulations! You are ready to begin the Fiber35 Diet. In this chapter, I will summarize the key parts of the program, and then we will put the knowledge you have learned into action.

Before I go any farther, I want to say a word about the key to your success. It is *you*. Of course you already knew that. You are the beginning, middle, and end of the story of success you are about to write. First of all, I want to congratulate you for having the courage to take back control of your weight and your health.

Today, we are surrounded by unhealthy "food" products that first entice us, then addict us, and finally kill us. We live in a time when we have to protect our health by resisting tremendous temptations—from supermarkets to ball games to the fast-food restaurants that stand on nearly every street corner in America. In essence, choosing to eat for optimum weight and health is like choosing not to smoke while growing up in a house full of smokers.

But you can do it. You now know how. The question is: why did you decide to lose weight? For all of us reading this book, there are old habits that we will have to leave behind, and new habits that need to be developed. This takes resolve, discipline, and the ability to overcome short-term temptation. For some of us, food is an emotional support system. And if you fall into that category, I know how much courage it takes to begin a new life, with a new relationship to food. For everyone, I would offer this word of advice. In order to succeed, you need to define your motivation. Why do you want to lose weight? Write it down. Write it here. Take your time with it. This is your mission statement. This is a letter to yourself that you reread to help yourself overcome moments of doubt.

YOUR PERSONAL MISSION STATEMENT

You'll find a page at the back of the book in Appendix A where you can copy this statement. Tear it out and make copies of it. Put one on your refrigerator; carry one in your wallet or purse; and place one next to your bed and read it before you go to sleep and when you wake up.

Ultimately, with the Fiber35 Diet, you are giving yourself the greatest gift there is—true wealth, which is your health. That is exactly how I view my own Fiber35 lifestyle.

Let's get started.

The three Fiber35 Diet factors you are going to put into action are:

1. **Putting together your high-fiber meal plan**

   Phase One: Accelerated Weight Loss
   Phase Two: Moderate Weight Loss
   Phase Three: Optimum Weight Maintenance for Life

2. **Incorporating metabolic boosters**

3. **Incorporating supplements**

PUTTING TOGETHER YOUR HIGH-FIBER MEAL PLAN

As you already know, there are three phases to the program. During the first two phases, you will reduce your calories to achieve your weight loss goal. In the third phase, you will eat a normal amount of calories and maintain your optimum weight. The following is your program summary.

Program Summary

	Phase 1	Phase 2	Phase 3
Time in Phase	2 to 4 weeks	Until You Reach Your Goal	Ongoing
Calorie Reduction	1,000 or fewer (no fewer than 1,200/day)	500 or fewer (no fewer than 1,200/day)	Amount to Maintain Your Desired Weight
Metabolic Boosters	5 to 7 (each day)	4 to 6 (each day)	3 to 4 (each day)
Daily Fiber	At least 35 grams	At least 35 grams	At least 35 grams

Throughout each phase, you will eat for optimum nutrition by choosing those foods outlined in the previous chapter. This means eating plenty of good carbs (fruits, vegetables, and whole grains) while avoiding the bad carbs (refined flours and sugars); eating plenty of good oils while avoiding the bad oils; and eating plenty of lean protein while avoiding fatty meats. Don't forget that you'll find samples of weekly meal planners—one for each phase of the Fiber35 Diet—in Chapter 15 to help guide you through choosing your daily menus as you proceed through the program. Chapter 15 also includes a shopping list and notes on where to find specialty items. In Appendix B you'll also find a blank daily journal page that you can tear out, copy, and use to help tally your total caloric and fiber intake for the day.

The initial step in putting together your meal plan for each of the phases is determining your caloric needs. In Chapter 4, you should have determined this factor. (If you skipped over that material and if you still don't want to do the math, you can just skim this section. However, I highly recommend calculating your daily caloric needs and completing the exercises here. Seeing the numbers on paper will help motivate you and keep you on track through the diet's phases.)

Let's now utilize that information.

Weight Loss Goal

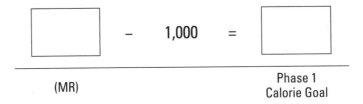

Enter your predetermined calories to maintain your current weight (otherwise called your metabolic rate, or MR).

*Reduce this number by 1,000 calories for Phase One.

Phase One: Accelerated Weight Loss

Remember: you will stay in Phase One for up to a month. I suggest you remain in this phase for at least two weeks.

Below is a sample day of your eating plan in Phase One. Note that this is based on a beginning caloric need of 2,200 calories. In Phase One, your caloric intake will be based on your predetermined caloric needs minus 1,000 calories. Example: metabolic rate of 2,200 minus 1,000 equals 1,200 calories a day.

Remember: don't go under 1,200 calories a day. For example, if a woman had a starting caloric need of 2,000, she would subtract only 800 calories for Phase One instead of 1,000, so as not to reduce her caloric intake below 1,200.

You may want to get an idea of how many calories to allow for each meal. In the following sample, I have 250 calories for breakfast and lunch and 400 calories for dinner, with 100 calories for each snack, equaling a total of 1,200 for the day. You can switch around any meals you wish. For example, it is OK to eat a lunch meal for breakfast or a dinner meal for lunch. Just make sure you track your total calories and fiber daily. It is also acceptable to eat out if you wish (some guidelines are presented on page 91). Try to find meals that allow you to meet your fiber and calorie goals for the day.

You can spread the fiber requirement out for the day just as you would your calories, making sure that you get 35 or more grams of fiber daily. You can boost the fiber of any meal by using the sprinkle table fiber or fiber wafers suggested in Chapter 10. The minimum amount of fiber per day is 35 grams, but 40–45 grams would be even better.

A Day in Phase One

Food	Calories	Fiber
Breakfast: fiber/protein shake drink* mixed with water and ½ cup frozen fruit or 4 ounces almond milk plus 4 ounces of water	250	10
Snack: ½ fiber/protein snack bar or fiber/protein snack from suggested snack list	100	5
Lunch: fiber/protein shake drink mixed with water and ½ cup frozen fruit or 4 ounces almond milk plus 4 ounces of water or meal containing fiber and protein (salad with chicken)	250	10
Snack: ½ fiber/protein snack bar or fiber/protein snack from suggested snack list	100	5
Dinner: meal containing fiber and protein (salmon and vegetables)	400	10
Snack: fiber/protein snack from the suggested snack list	100	5
Total:	1,200	45
Fiber flush effect (45 grams fiber × 7 calories)**	− 315	
Net calories	885	

* You can use a shake mix or ready-to-drink shakes. You will find shake recipes in Chapter 14. I recommend blending a shake at home for breakfast and taking a ready-to-drink shake to work for lunch, along with your snacks. In Phase One, a 175-pound woman, for example, will frequently consume fiber/protein shakes for breakfast and fiber/protein snack bars. Shakes and bars make it easy to control your calories and portion sizes. This is more critical in Phase One. The shakes and snack bars are also easy to prepare and convenient to take to work.

** Fiber flush effect: Keep in mind that with the fiber flush effect or fecal energy excretion, you excrete in your stool 7 calories for every gram of fiber you consume. At the end of the day, by taking this into account you will be able to calculate your net calories for the day—the calories your body has absorbed and will actually use.

Timing Your Meals and Snacks

As you can see from the sample, you will be eating frequently throughout the day. Following is the recommended eating plan.

Time	Meal / Snack
7:00 a.m.	Breakfast: shake or meal
10:00 a.m.	Snack
12:00 p.m.	Lunch: shake or meal
3:00 p.m.	Snack
6:00 p.m.	Dinner
7:30 p.m.	Snack

7:30 p.m. Cutoff Time

Do not eat past 7:30 at night, as this may slow your weight loss. You should allow several hours between your last meal or snack and your bedtime.

Food Restrictions in Phase One

During Phase One of the Fiber35 Plan, you need to restrict dairy to low-fat or no-fat. As you progress into Phase Two, you can incorporate full-fat dairy. Avoid alcohol whenever possible. If you are attending a social event or special occasion and want to partake of an alcoholic drink, you must calculate it into your calories for the day. For example, a 5-ounce glass of red wine is about 100 calories. During Phase One, avoid or limit starchy-type vegetables, such as potatoes, yams, and carrots. Try to limit caffeine, as it has been shown to raise blood sugar levels. If you are a coffee drinker, try switching to green tea, which has less caffeine.

Floater Meals

A floater meal is one in which you substitute a meal for a shake during the week. Any time you are having a really hard time consuming another shake, eat a meal. The key to this program is that if you need a meal, I never want you to feel you are cheating or failing by having one "when you shouldn't." Fiber35 is a lifetime plan for optimum weight and health. Floater meals may slow down the pace of your weight loss, but truly, the slowdown is negligible when you consider the fact that this is your lifetime plan. If your goal is to lose 50 pounds, who cares if it takes an extra week? Use your floater meals when the need arises!

Tips for Phase One

Reminder: refer to Chapter 15 for a suggested weekly meal plan for Phase One.

- **Do not consume fewer than 1,200 calories each day.**

- **Keep a journal of everything you eat and drink to make sure you're staying within your targeted number of calories for the day (use the journal template I've provided in Appendix B).**

- **Eat five to six times each day.**

- **Use five to seven metabolic boosters each day (described below, and at length in Chapter 7).**

- **Consume a minimum of 35 grams of fiber per day.**

- **Increase your fiber consumption to 45 to 50 grams if desired.**

- **Drink at least half your body weight in ounces of water daily. Example: If you weight 150 pounds, drink 75 ounces of water each day.**

- **Consider taking a fiber supplement before your meals to help increase feelings of fullness and prevent overeating.**

Phase Two: Moderate Weight Loss

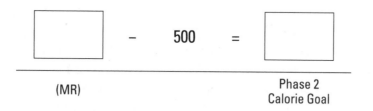

$$\boxed{} \quad - \quad 500 \quad = \quad \boxed{}$$

(MR)   Phase 2
                                        Calorie Goal

Remember: you will remain in Phase Two until you reach your weight loss goal.

Following is a sample day of your eating plan in Phase Two. This is based on the same beginning caloric need as in Phase One: 2,200 calories. In Phase Two, your caloric intake will be based on your predetermined caloric need minus 500 calories. For example, 2,200 minus 500 equals 1,700 calories a day. Again, as noted in Phase One, don't go under 1,200 calories per day. The same guidelines about switching meals and eating out apply in Phase Two.

In Phase Two, as in Phase One, you can divvy up your individual caloric needs throughout the day's snacks and meals, as well as the fiber requirements. To boost the fiber of any meal, remember to use sprinkle table fiber or fiber wafers.

Your main goal in Phase Two is to get at least 35 grams of fiber daily, but 40 to 45 grams will be even better and will enhance your weight loss.

A Day in Phase Two

Food	Calories	Fiber
Breakfast: fiber/protein shake drink* mixed with water or almond milk and ½ cup frozen fruit	250	10
Snack: 1 fiber/protein snack bar or fiber/protein snack from suggested snack list	200	5
Lunch: meal containing fiber and protein (salad with chicken)	500	10
Snack: fiber/protein snack from the suggested snack list	150	5
Dinner: meal containing fiber and protein (salmon and vegetables)	500	10
Snack: fiber/protein snack from the suggested snack list	100	5
Total:	1700	45
Fiber flush effect (45 grams fiber × 7 calories)**	– 315	
Net calories	1385	

* Note: There is only one meal during the day for which you would substitute a shake, as compared with Phase One. If you prefer, you can continue to use two shakes per day, or use a shake as one of your snacks.

** The fiber flush effect still applies here and will allow you to subtract 7 calories for each gram of fiber consumed. At the end of the day, you will be able to calculate your net calories for the day—the calories your body has absorbed and will actually use.

Timing Your Meals and Snacks

You will continue to scatter your meals and snacks throughout the day, using the same eating plan as in Phase One, and avoid eating after 7:30 p.m.

Food Restrictions in Phase Two

During Phase Two of the Fiber35 plan, you are able to include full-fat dairy foods and some starchy vegetables. Continue to avoid alcohol whenever possible. Again, if you are attending a social event or special occasion and want to partake of an alcoholic drink, you must calculate it into your calories for the day. Use the same guidelines for caffeine as you did in Phase One.

Floater Meals

Floater meals, as described above, do not apply in Phase Two, because you are already eating at least two full meals daily.

Tips for Phase Two

Reminder: refer to Chapter 15 for a suggested weekly meal plan for Phase Two.

- **Do not consume fewer than 1,200 calories each day.**

- **Keep a journal of everything you eat and drink just as you did in Phase One using a copy of the journal entry page in Appendix B.**

- **Eat five to six times each day.**

- **Use four to six metabolic boosters each day.**

- **Consume a minimum of 35 grams of fiber per day.**

- **Increase your fiber consumption to 45 to 60 grams if desired.**

- **Drink at least half your body weight in ounces of water daily.**

- **Consider taking fiber before each meal to help increase feelings of fullness and prevent overeating.**

Phase Three: Weight Maintenance

In Phase Three, you are in Fiber35 for Life. This is when the diet becomes a lifestyle. You are now eating three meals per day, and snacking three additional times, on the basis of your individual caloric needs. You are no longer reducing your calorie intake but are continuing to eat 35 to 45 grams of fiber-rich foods daily, utilizing the Optimum Nutrition Food Choices as outlined in Chapter 5. In this phase, you will eat slightly larger meals than you did in the earlier phases. You can drink fewer shakes and consume larger portions of desserts.

In Phase Three, your goal is to manage your daily caloric intake in order to maintain your ideal weight. You will determine your new personal daily calorie goal by recalculating your estimated metabolic rate (MR) on the basis of your new weight. That calculation is shown below.

Step 1: Calculate Resting Calories (Metabolic Rate Expressed as "Resting Calories")

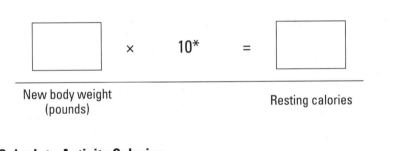

New body weight (pounds)   Resting calories

Step 2: Calculate Activity Calories

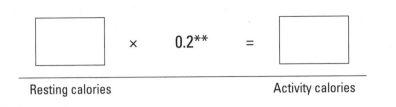

Resting calories   Activity calories

Step 3: Add Resting Calories and Activity Calories

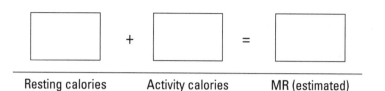

| Resting calories | Activity calories | MR (estimated) |

* Use 10 for women and 11 for men.

** Use 0.2 if you are inactive, 0.3 if you are somewhat active and 0.4 if you are moderately active.

Let's take as an example a 175-pound woman who lost 25 pounds in Phase One and Phase Two. Her original estimated metabolic rate was 2,100 calories per day (175 × 10 = 1,750; 1,750 × 0.2 = 350, 1,750 + 350 = 2,100 calories per day). In Phase Three, her new daily goal is to consume as many calories as she needs to match her new MR. That would be approximately 1,800 calories each day (150 × 10 = 1,500; 1,500 × 0.2 = 300, 1,500 + 300 = 1,800 calories per day). She can stay in Phase Three as long as she maintains her desired ideal weight. By continuing to consume 35 grams of fiber daily, she will find it easier to maintain this weight. The fiber will help her stay full during the day, and the fiber flush effect will continue to eliminate additional calories.

You will want to monitor your weight closely in the coming months. I highly recommend that you continue to record your calorie and fiber intake daily. Use the journal entry template I've provided in Appendix B; make copies of it and fill one out every day! By doing so, you'll be able to see if you are too high on calories or too low on fiber, and you will be able to adjust your diet accordingly. There's no better way to know exactly how much you're eating than to keep track of what you put into your mouth. We all tend to underestimate how much we eat unless we're writing it down!

The estimated metabolic rate is only an estimate of the calories and fiber you need. If you find that your weight is increasing slightly, lower your total caloric intake, increase your metabolic boosters, and increase your daily intake of fiber. Full descriptions of these metabolic boosters are coming up. Try to get at least three to four metabolic boosters each day, because these will help keep your metabolic rate elevated and make it easier to maintain the ideal weight you have achieved.

If you go off the plan at any time, and gain more weight, don't worry. Just go back to Phase One or Phase Two to return to your optimum weight, and then move into Phase Three.

Tips for Phase Three

- Keep a journal of everything you eat and drink.

- Eat five to six times each day.

- Use three to four metabolic boosters each day.

- Consume a minimum of 35 grams of fiber daily.

- Increase your fiber consumption to 45 to 60 grams if desired.

- Drink at least half your body weight in ounces of water daily.

- Take fiber before each meal to help increase your sense of fullness.

Reminder: refer to Chapter 15 for a suggested weekly meal plan for Phase Three.

INCORPORATING METABOLIC BOOSTERS

During all three phases of the Fiber35 Diet Plan, it's important to implement as many of the metabolic boosters as you can. I do realize there may be one or two that you might not succeed in using consistently, and that is why I've provided seven. Each of you may be different regarding which specific metabolic boosters you find easiest to implement consistently.

I'll be going into great detail about each of these seven metabolic boosters in Chapter 7, but let me give you an introduction to them here.

Metabolic Booster 1—Frequent Eating

Guess what—this is already built into the Fiber35 way of eating. In following the meal plans as outlined above, you will be eating six times a day. Count this one as a freebie!

Metabolic Booster 2—Muscle Boosting

Chapter 8 details a strength training system using resistance bands. There is a twenty-minute routine, as well as a forty-minute routine. Try to do the twenty-minute routine, alternating the upper and lower body, four to five times a week. If you do the forty-minute full-body routine, aim to do it three times a week. (See Resource Directory for sources of resistance bands.)

Metabolic Booster 3—Aerobic Exercise

Chapter 8 also details the suggested cardio exercises. Incorporate a cardio exercise such as power walking on a treadmill three times a week. Either alternate days with the resistance band routines or do the routines on same day (cardio in the morning and resistance bands in the evening).

For more information and images of exercising with the resistance band, please go to www.fiber35diet.com.

Metabolic Booster 4—Water, Water, Water

Throughout the day, preferably between meals, drink half your body weight in ounces of clean, purified water. (The amount is determined by dividing your body weight—using pounds rather than kilograms—by two.) For example, a 160-pound person would need to drink 80 ounces of water daily. If you do not like drinking plain water, the menu chapter has some suggestions about how to get water from other tasty beverages. Caffeinated drinks do not count as part of your daily water intake. When you are increasing fiber, it's also important to increase your water intake.

Metabolic Booster 5—Sleep

I know how hard it can be sometimes, but try to get eight full hours of sleep each night. Sleep deprivation accumulates. If you are short on your eight hours one or more nights during the week, try to make up for the deficit on the weekend. Use a natural sleep aid when necessary (see page 105).

Metabolic Booster 6—Sauna

Try to enjoy a sauna two to three times a week in the privacy of your home, using a personal infrared sauna. As you'll soon learn in Chapter 7, thirty minutes in a sauna is like running a 5-mile race. (See Resource Directory for a source of personal infrared saunas.)

Metabolic Booster 7—Detox

Chapter 9 details the effect toxins have on your efforts to lose weight. I'll explain how you can utilize a herbal detoxification program at the beginning of the Fiber35 Diet Plan. You can continue to detox two to three times per year. The sauna will also help to detoxify your body.

INCORPORATING SUPPLEMENTS

Chapter 10 will detail specific supplements that can be helpful in your Fiber35 Diet Plan. It's not necessary to take every supplement. Many supplements are optional, depending on your situation.

The health maintenance supplements, omega-3 fatty acids, and multivitamin/mineral formula should be taken by everyone, every day, regardless of weight.

The fiber supplements can be utilized as needed in order to obtain 35 to 45 grams of fiber daily. If you find you are short on fiber toward the end of the day, take a scoop of the bulk fiber supplement or eat a chewable fiber wafer.

Chew fiber supplements before a meal.

HOW TO AVOID PROBLEMS WHEN YOU ARE INCREASING FIBER

When you are increasing your daily intake of dietary fiber, remember to consume a variety of soluble and insoluble fiber foods including fruits, vegetables, and whole grain breads and cereals. You may temporarily experience some gas or bloating when you increase the amount of fiber in your diet too quickly. This is particularly true if you attempt to increase the fiber in your diet from only a few food types. For example, if you increase your consumption of cereal or breads dramatically, you could have some intestinal discomfort. It's better to eat a variety of high-fiber foods from many natural sources. If you experience too much gas and bloating, you can reduce the amount of fiber you are eating for a few days and then gradually continue to increase your fiber intake until you achieve your goals.

It bears repeating that you should be sure to consume plenty water or liquids every day. If you are taking powdered fiber supplements, be aware that they can become thick and difficult to swallow. Make sure to mix them in plenty of water, juice, or fluid of your choice, and drink them soon after mixing. There are also many new fiber supplements that dissolve clearly in water. These are mostly soluble fiber powders that are easy to mix and drink. Your goal is to increase the level of fiber in your diet gradually and maintain this level for the rest of your life.

TIPS ON EATING OUT

No, you don't have to lock yourself up at home until you've reached your weight loss goal. It's perfectly fine to eat out in each phase of the Fiber35 Diet. Just make sure to count that meal as one of your full meals during the day if you're in the first or second phase. No matter which phase you're in, be careful to select foods that are consistent with the diet guidelines. That said, here are some additional guidelines:

- Choose a protein and vegetable sides, or a salad.

- Order grilled, not fried, protein and stay away from rich gravies.

- If possible, use oil and vinegar as your salad dressing, or use a low-calorie dressing.

- Ask the waiter not to bring bread to the table.

- Choose extra-virgin olive oil.

- Have a small protein-source snack before going out to eat or to a party. For example, try a few slices of turkey on whole-grain bread with a slice of reduced-fat cheddar cheese. Or if dairy works for you, try a serving of low-fat cottage cheese.

- Order a cup of clear broth as an appetizer, as this will fill you up before the entrée.

- Do not be afraid to ask specific questions about the menu.

- Do not be afraid to special-order a meal to be cooked differently.

- Stay away from white potatoes and white rice.

- Ask for dressings and sauces on the side. Use a fork to drizzle them over food, instead of pouring them.

- If you are going to a fast-food restaurant, order a grilled chicken breast sandwich or a salad with chicken. Skip the dressing or order low-cal.

- If you must eat a dessert, use the three-bite rule: take three bites and then ask the waiter to take it away.

Getting Started with the Fiber35 Diet

- **These meal plans, along with the metabolic boosters and the suggested supplements, will enable you to lose the desired amount of weight steadily and keep it off for life.**

- **The three Fiber35 Diet factors you are going to put into action are:**

    Putting together your high-fiber meal plan

    - Phase One—accelerated weight loss
    - Phase Two—moderate weight loss
    - Phase Three—weight maintenance

    Incorporating metabolic boosters

    Incorporating supplements

THE FIBER35 DIET METABOLIC BOOSTERS

Shaving calories from your daily needs will greatly assist you in meeting your weight loss goal, but it's only half of the program. The other half, known as the Fiber35 Diet Metabolic Boosters, will help ensure that you maximize your weight loss by supporting your metabolism during and after each weight loss phase.

THE SEVEN COMPONENTS

Seven may seem like a lot of components to keep track of, but don't panic; they are actually quite easy to incorporate into your plan. Let's review again what the seven metabolic boosters are:

1. **Frequent eating (5 or 6 times daily)**

2. **Muscle boosting**

3. **Aerobic exercise**

4. **Water, water, water**

5. **Eight hours of sleep per night**

6. **Sauna**

7. **Detox**

I cannot overemphasize how important these boosters are to your success in losing weight. When they are combined with the Fiber35 Diet, they will counteract the reason why most diets fail.

The Fiber35 Diet's Fail-Safe Secret

Earlier, we touched on the concept of your metabolism and the physiological double whammy—the process that occurs when you reduce calories and your body starts working against your efforts to achieve your weight loss goal. I also like to call this the "double-hunger-whammy." While you see restricting calories as the way to lose weight, your body interprets this as a threat of starvation. In response, a rush of hunger signals entice you to eat more; and at the same time, your metabolism slows down to conserve the lower number of calories you are eating. This puts you in a very difficult position. Suddenly, you find yourself ravenous, and everything you put into your mouth—even good food—is likely to be stored as fat, as if you were living in the Stone Age and your body didn't know when you'd get your next meal.

These are two physiological defense mechanisms you need for survival, but obviously not for weight loss. And this is the main reason why most diets that severely restrict calories fail.

Let's say you decide you want to lose weight. You set a goal of losing 10 pounds by reducing calories. You skip breakfast, drink a shake for lunch, munch on celery in the afternoon, and eat a small dinner in the evening. The first few days are tough, but you are determined to persevere. After a week, you have lost 3 pounds. You are constantly hungry—and fantasizing about food—and you find the second week even more of a struggle. You combat your hunger signals all day long, telling yourself that if you can get through the diet, you'll feel and look great. By the end of the second week, you have lost a total of 5 pounds. You are still hungry all day long, your willpower is being tested more and more; but you stick to your plan, and two weeks later you have reached your goal of losing 10 pounds. Fantastic! Then, thirty days later, lo and behold, not only did you regain the 10 pounds you lost, but you also added an extra 5 pounds. Why?

During the month of weight loss, unbeknownst to you, your metabolism slowed down considerably. Because you were eating less, you tricked your body into thinking it needed less fuel to function. Not only that, but because you were not getting enough water, vitamins, minerals, amino acids, and complex carbohydrates, your body began burning protein for energy, and much of your weight loss ended up being water and muscle (lean body mass) instead of your target—fat. So you lost 10 pounds, but in doing so, you unknowingly set yourself up for the yo-yo effect.

Here's what happened, metabolically. After losing the 10 pounds, you stopped the diet and were hungrier than ever. So you started eating, and you ate more than you normally ate before you went on the diet. Why? Because your body sent incredibly powerful hunger signals to "stop the starvation." Even worse, because you were not using the metabolic boosters I am about to teach you, your metabolism slowed down to a snail's pace during your thirty-day crash diet. The result? You came out of the diet burning fewer calories than you were burning before you went on the diet. When you do the math—you're eating more now and burning less—you can see how the pounds can come back quickly. And you can blame the extra 5 pounds on your metabolism, which had to downshift when you put your body into starvation mode. As soon as you began to eat again, more of the calories were converted to fat.

Believe me, we have all been there. But don't worry. With the Fiber35 Diet, this is not going to happen—for several reasons. First, the Fiber35 Diet teaches you a lifelong formula that allows you to eat all day long without bingeing when your weight loss phases are completed. The fiber in your diet will help control your cravings for food, so that when the weight loss phases are over, you will not feel a surge of hunger. Second, the Fiber35 Diet formula for a successful calorie reduction that doesn't sabotage your metabolism is not complicated. And third, the Fiber35 Diet Metabolic Boosters, as part of the Fiber35Diet, will help you maintain your metabolism while you restrict your calories, helping to keep your calorie-burning fire going even though you are eating less. You'll also lose predominantly fat, not water or muscle.

What's more, when you come out of Phase Two, you won't go back to unhealthy eating habits. You'll use my Fiber35 Diet for Life Plan and continue to nourish your body with my optimum nutrition food choices. How hard does that sound? Just wait until you see how good you'll *feel*. You'll never want to go back to the way you've been eating.

DON'T FORGET ABOUT THE METABOLIC EFFECT OF FIBER

A high-fiber diet positively influences your metabolic rate. In a large collaborative study spanning more than two years, researchers found that a very low-fat, reduced-calorie diet made people feel tired, cold, and hungry; however, a high-fiber diet left them more energetic and refreshed while protecting their cardiovascular systems. The extra calories burned by the metabolic effect of a high-fiber diet, according to these scientists, could result in removing several extra pounds a year. In their calculations the high-fiber effect equaled the calories used up by walking about a mile a day—80 calories daily. The diet also improved insulin sensitivity in the experimental group twice as much as in a group that ate merely a low-fat diet.[1]

GETTING TO KNOW YOUR METABOLISM BOOSTERS

We've been talking about metabolism since the start of this book. Simply put, your metabolism, also known as your metabolic rate, is the rate at which you burn calories to run all of your bodily functions. When you think, walk, digest food, or pump blood throughout your body, you are burning calories. Even when you sleep, you are burning calories. The faster your metabolism, the more calories you burn.

Literally every cell in your body requires energy to carry out its particular job. Some areas of the body burn more calories to maintain and operate themselves than others. For example, muscle tissue requires a lot of energy to maintain itself, so the more muscle you have, the higher your metabolism runs to keep your muscles in working order and the more calories you naturally burn.

It's understandable that the faster your metabolism, the more calories you burn, and the more food you need to eat to maintain your weight. You probably know some skinny friend who eats like a horse but doesn't gain any weight. The reason is probably that his or her metabolic rate is higher than yours. You may also have tried to lose weight before and struggled even though you reduced your calories. The reason is probably your metabolic rate. There are several factors that affect your metabolic rate—age, gender, height, and genetics, to name a few. Some people, genetically, have a faster metabolism—like your skinny friend who eats so much—but many others are not this lucky.

Fortunately, you can supercharge your metabolism with the Fiber35 Diet Metabolic Boosters. Let's get to know more about each of these seven components.

Metabolic Booster 1: Frequent Eating

You may be doing a double take right now. How could I suggest that in order to lose weight, you need to eat frequently. Well, you've read this right. When I said frequently, I meant five or six times a day. Why is that?

The concept is called dietary thermogenesis—the energy our bodies require to digest food. Digestion is a very energy-intensive process. It takes work to convert, say, barbecued chicken into the macronutrients (protein, carbohydrates, fat) and micronutrients that your body can actually utilize for energy. You can think of this as a process, like refining oil into usable gasoline to run your car. The refinery must burn energy to convert oil into the fuel you pump into your car at the gas station.

Every time you eat, you have to burn calories in order to digest your food and unlock the energy within your meal. And guess what—eating increases your metabolic rate. In fact, studies have shown that during the eating process, your metabolism increases as much as 30 percent, and this effect lasts up to three hours after you have finished eating. Fasting, on the other hand, lowers your metabolic rate. The reason so many diets fail is that meals are skipped, or long periods of time elapse between meals, and this slows down your metabolism and decreases the rate at which you burn calories.

The key to maximizing weight loss when you restrict calories is to continually fire up your metabolism through dietary thermogenesis. How? By eating smaller portions every two to three hours or so, you increase the frequency with which your metabolism is fired up to fuel the digestive process. If your metabolism is increased for as long as three hours after eating, and you are eating every two to three hours, you will consistently engage your dietary thermogenesis process. This dietary thermogenesis response is triggered by all types of nutrients: fat, carbs, and protein. Therefore, a very important factor in all phases of the Fiber35 Diet is to eat every two to three hours. You might be thinking that this is going to take a lot of work, but in reality it does not. There are twenty-four hours in a day, and you will scatter your meals and snacks over the course of about twelve hours. So if you eat breakfast at 7 a.m., and then eat every two to three hours thereafter, you will be done with your last snack at 7:30 p.m. You will then have eaten five or six times during the day, keeping your dietary thermogenesis engaged, and thus increasing your metabolism. Very little food preparation is involved.

Metabolic Booster 2: Muscle Boosting

Lean muscle mass is largely responsible for your rate of metabolism. Muscle cells are about eight times more metabolically demanding than fat cells. Muscle is more metabolically active than fat because muscle tissue is extremely active even when you are resting. For example, when you are surfing the Web, you probably consider yourself to be resting, but even the smallest muscular movements require energy expenditure by the body. Fat, by contrast, is relatively inactive from a metabolic perspective, and just sits there.

The greater your ratio of lean body mass is to fat, the faster your metabolism runs and the more calories you burn. If you want to increase your metabolic rate, you need to increase your lean body mass. And if you want to maintain your metabolic rate while restricting your calories and losing weight, you need to maintain your lean muscle mass. Of the seven metabolic boosters, muscle boosting is the most important.

How do you build and maintain your lean body mass? By strength training! Strength training can increase metabolic rate by as much as 15 percent. This increase is enormously helpful for weight loss and long-term weight control. Now you might be thinking: I have never done any form of strength training, and I don't know how to do it. Don't worry; it's easy to learn. All you need to do is follow the Fiber35 Diet two twenty-minute workouts provided in Chapter 8. I call this the Fiber35 Diet Strength-Training System (it uses resistance bands), and I highly recommend that you perform a workout two to four times per week. Women reading this may be thinking that they don't want to look muscular. You won't, but you will look toned, and in becoming so, you will probably burn more calories than you ever have burned before. Strength training has numerous other benefits as well. It helps support strong bones, wards off osteoporosis, and has been shown to reduce the signs and symptoms of certain diseases and chronic conditions such as arthritis, diabetes, obesity, back pain, and depression.

By doing the Fiber35 Diet Strength-Training System, you are going to help maintain and gain lean body mass. There's no better way to make your muscles strong and achieve a higher amount of calorie-burning lean muscle mass. Combined with the right carbohydrates, this system can fuel your muscles and maintain lean body mass at any age.

Nutritional Supplement Tip: Lean Muscle Mass Formula

To enhance the increase in lean muscle mass you'll build through my strength training program, you may use a nutritional supplement that contains non-stimulatory natural ingredients that will further assist you. Visit your local health food store and ask for help in choosing the right formula (also refer to the Resource Directory). Look for three key ingredients: banaba extract, conjugated linoleic acid (CLA), and medium-chain triglycerides (MCTs).[2] Banaba, an extract from a Philippine herb, affects lean muscle mass indirectly by increasing insulin sensitivity. With increased insulin sensitivity, fat is burned more efficiently, creating a favorable ratio of fat to lean muscle.

Conjugated linoleic acid is a form of the essential fatty acid linoleic acid, found primarily in animal foods. Numerous studies on humans and animals have confirmed that CLA decreases abdominal fat and enhances muscle growth. It has the added benefit of increasing metabolic rate, and, like banaba, may have the long-term effect of increasing insulin sensitivity and glycemic control, thus helping weight management. It's important to realize that CLA promotes fat loss, not necessarily weight loss. One study found that when dieters resumed normal eating and regained weight, those taking CLA were more likely to gain muscle than fat. It's further been established that the effectiveness of CLA in reducing fat mass and increasing lean muscle is improved with regular exercise.

Studies have also shown that a diet rich in medium-chain triglycerides (MCTs), which are a class of fatty acids typically derived from lauric oils (e.g., coconut and palm kernel oil), results in a greater loss of fatty tissue than a diet composed largely of the more commonly consumed long-chain fatty acids. Because of their shorter chain, MCTs are more easily digested, have a slightly lower calorie content than other fats, and may increase calorie burning compared with other fats. They also stimulate metabolism, enhance the action of insulin, and help you feel full faster.

Metabolic Booster 3: Aerobic Exercise

Aerobic exercise significantly boosts your metabolism. Although it is possible to lose weight without exercising, a regular exercise routine—three times per week for at least thirty minutes per session—will greatly accelerate your weight loss. Most important, by exercising, you will receive all the associated health benefits that come along with exercise. Foremost, it is a boon to the cardiovascular system.

Aerobic exercise helps you to lose weight and boosts your metabolism in three ways. First, it heightens your metabolism during your exercise period and burns a significant number of extra calories. A typical forty-five-minute aerobic exercise period burns 350 extra calories. If you exercise three times per week for forty-five minutes each time, you will burn 1,050 calories during your workouts. Over a month's time, that's 4,200 calories, or more than 1 pound. Over a year, that's an extra 12 pounds.

Second, if the exercise is high-intensity (meaning that it causes a significant increase in your heart rate and respiration), your metabolism will remain elevated for an extended period of time, so that you will continue to burn calories at an accelerated rate after you have stopped exercising.

Third, aerobic exercise maintains lean muscle mass, which is crucial during your weight loss phase. Your objective is to lose fat, not muscle. Some aerobic exercises actually increase lean muscle mass, but many do not. For this reason, aerobic exercise should be done in combination with strength training, so that you are increasing your lean muscle mass while getting the immediate calorie-burning benefit of the aerobic exercise.

Although strength training can certainly be done at a pace that is considered aerobic, in most cases it's anaerobic. Strength training can certainly elevate your heart rate and help you burn extra calories; but more important, it increases lean muscle mass, which increases your metabolic rate to help you burn more calories twenty-four hours a day. By mixing aerobic activity with strength training, you give yourself the maximum benefit.

The key to your aerobic exercise program is to find one or two exercises you enjoy, since you'll be more apt to do them. You should exercise three times per week for at least thirty minutes per session. Below is a chart that shows various exercises and how many calories you will burn in a one-hour session.

Calories Burned by 1 Hour of Exercise

Exercise	Calories Burned
Aerobics, general	422
Aerobics, low-impact	352
Aerobics, high-impact	493
Bicycling, leisurely, <10 mph	281
Bicycling, moderate, 10–14 mph	563
Bicycling, vigorous, 14–16 mph	704
Dancing, aerobic, general	422
Gardening, moderate activity	352
Golf, walking (no cart)	281
Health club exercise, general	387
Jogging 5 mph (12-minute mile) or less	493
Rowing, stationary, light effort	493
Rowing, stationary, moderate effort	598
Rowing, stationary, vigorous	844
Running, 7 mph (8.5-minute mile)	809
Running, 8.6 mph (7-minute mile)	985
Running, all-out 10 mph (6-minute mile)	1126
Skating, ice, general	387
Stair/treadmill, general	422
Stretching, hatha yoga	281
Swimming laps, freestyle-moderate	563
Swimming laps, freestyle, fast	704
Tai chi	281
Walking, 2 mph, slow pace	176
Walking, 3 mph, moderate pace	246
Walking, 4 mph, very brisk pace	281
Weight lifting, light/moderate	211
Weight lifting, heavy	422

Nutritional Supplement Tip: Thermogenic Formula

Exercise alone can boost your metabolism by enhancing thermogenesis (heat production in the body), but this effect can be assisted by a well-formulated thermogenic nutritional supplement. Such an energy-boosting formula would ideally contain a variety of natural substances that support the activity of the thyroid gland (which regulates metabolism), increase the burning of fat, regulate blood sugar and insulin levels, and suppress appetite. Again, a local health food store that specializes in supplements should be able to help you find the right one. You should also discuss your supplements with your physician when you consult with him or her prior to starting the fitness regimen. Ingredients to look for in a thermogenic formula include iodine, tyrosine, green tea extract, banaba, and bitter orange peel extract.

The mineral iodine and the amino acid tyrosine are important thyroid regulators. Abnormalities of iodine metabolism, which can result in thyroid disease and obesity, can be prevented through ingestion of kelp, a whole food supplement that provides iodine to support the thyroid gland and balance metabolism. As a direct precursor to the thyroid hormone thyroxine, tyrosine is an important ingredient in weight loss, one that also helps regulate appetite.

Green tea extract has garnered lots of acclaim in recent years following studies that show its potential effect in enhancing metabolism and aiding fat oxidation. Studies also show that it can help control body weight by helping to reduce blood fats—cholesterol—as well as aiding in blood sugar balance.

Banaba, in addition to being found in lean muscle mass formulas, may also help regulate blood sugar levels. That is why it's often found in thermogenic formulas.

Bitter orange peel extract contains compounds that help stimulate metabolism, as does the South American herb yerba mate, which also suppresses appetite. Other natural ingredients that may assist in weight loss include bamboo leaf extract and the natural brain chemical DMAE (short for dimethyl-amino-ethanol).

Note: You're going to get a lot of information on supplements in Chapter 10. However, you won't find specific instructions about how much of these supplements to take and when. You should share your intentions to begin a supplement program with your physician before you start, and I also highly recommend finding an educated and knowledgeable person to help you choose the right formula. Not all formulas are the same; and not all of them contain the same ingredients. Always follow recommended guidelines and label directions.

Metabolic Booster 4: Water, Water, Water

It's no secret that you need to drink eight or more glasses of water a day; after all, water is essential to every function of the body. But did you know that water helps you lose weight? Researchers in Germany measured the resting metabolic rate of fourteen men and women before and after they drank 16 ounces of water. After ten minutes, metabolism began to increase; and after forty minutes, the resting metabolic rate was as much as 30 percent higher. This boost in metabolism lasted for as much as an hour. But precisely why this happens is still not known.

While you restrict calories (and even when you don't), you should make absolutely sure that you drink a glass of water every hour or two, for a total of eight to twelve glasses per day. A good rule of thumb, which I mentioned earlier, is to drink half your weight in ounces each day. If you weigh 150 pounds, you should drink 75 ounces per day. This ensures that you provide more fuel for your metabolic fire, which keeps your calorie-burning machine humming. And keep in mind that drinking cold water can increase your metabolism even more than drinking room-temperature water because your body must expend more energy to warm cold water up to your normal body temperature.

There is something else that you should know about water. Many people mistake thirst for hunger. Instead of drinking enough water, they respond to their thirst as if it were hunger pangs, and eat instead. In essence, drinking plenty of water helps reduce the misperception of hunger, helping you eat less. And because water takes up so much volume in your stomach, it's a good idea to drink a tall glassful before you eat; this can help reduce the amount of food you consume at your meal. I recommend drinking a glass of water thirty minutes before eating a meal, to prepare the stomach for food. Then, during your meal, take small sips of water as you enjoy your food. You don't want to gulp too much water down as you eat, or all that water can dilute your stomach acid and cause digestive problems.

WATER WITH MEALS

Drink a glass of water about thirty minutes before eating, to prepare the stomach; then casually sip water during your meal. But don't drink too much while eating or you will dilute your stomach acid and potentially hamper digestion.

Metabolic Booster 5: Eight Hours of Sleep

If you sleep more, will you weigh less? The body of evidence that says *yes* continues to grow, proving that sleep could be just as important to maintaining ideal weight as what you eat and how much you exercise.

Our knowledge about the power of sleep has become clearer in recent years. In late 2004, studies began to emerge that showed a strong connection between one's sleep patterns and one's ability to lose weight, igniting a new public interest in sleep. Two groundbreaking studies in particular—one from the University of Chicago and the other from Stanford University—demonstrated the effects of sleep on the balance between two important hormones that tell you whether you are hungry or full.[3]

One of these hormones—leptin—is released by fat cells to indicate the level of fat stores available to the body. The other hormone—ghrelin—is released by the stomach to signal hunger. So leptin says, "Stop eating," whereas ghrelin says, "Feed me." When you are sleep-deprived, leptin levels are reduced and ghrelin levels increase. A lower leptin level tells your body that you do not have enough fat stored, and a higher ghrelin level tells your body that you are hungry. Together, they send signals to the brain that the body needs more energy, and the brain then creates signals that typically result in your storming the kitchen and eating a lot. Since those first studies, many others have been published that also show the damaging effects sleep deprivation can have on metabolism and one's ability to curb cravings. If you've ever had a hard time controlling cravings for sugary snacks and carbs after a bad night's sleep, you may be able to blame it on your lack of sleep and the resulting imbalance of appetite hormones rushing through you.

Aside from these hormonal factors, however, there's a practical relationship between sleep and weight loss that deserves note. Face it: when you don't get enough sleep, your energy is lower during the day. This can negatively influence two factors—food consumption and physical activity. When the body feels tired from a lack of sleep, it seeks to increase energy by consuming food. This is when cravings for salt, fat, and sugar hit hard. And when you are tired, you'll be likely to engage in less physical activity, further slowing down your metabolism.

The bottom line is that getting a full eight hours of sleep is critical to maintaining your metabolism—no matter in which phase of the diet you are. If possible, increase your sleep to nine hours in Phase One and Phase Two. I know that this much time is hard to find, but if you choose sleep over television or reading during these phases, your metabolism will thank you and your weight loss will improve.

NUTRITIONAL SUPPLEMENT TIP: NATURAL SLEEP AID

Many people today have difficulty falling asleep or sleeping through the night. Some opt for sleeping pills, which may help in the short term but pose many risks in the long term, including chemical or psychological dependency. Interestingly, one major conclusion from all the studies is that insomniacs are better off without sleeping pills than with them.

There are safe alternatives to sleeping pills, however. You can improve your ability to fall asleep and stay asleep by using a well-formulated nutritional supplement that features a combination of proven vitamin, mineral, herbal, and other natural ingredients to support your sleep cycle naturally and safely. Look for a formula that contains the ingredients described below. (Remember that with any supplement it's important to consult your physician before starting a regimen, especially if you take any prescription medication that could potentially conflict with ingredients in the supplement.)

Minerals in such a formula include calcium and magnesium, both of which have a calming effect on your brain. Magnesium deficiency has been shown to produce sleeplessness by altering electrical activity in the brain. Calcium helps convert the amino acid tryptophan to melatonin, a natural hormone that can make you sleepy. A formula that also contains a small amount of melatonin, which is naturally secreted by the pineal gland at night to help us sleep, can be particularly effective in regulating cycles of waking and sleeping. The addition of 5-HTP, a direct precursor to the feel-good brain chemical serotonin, can help, too. Serotonin not only is known to enhance sleep but also helps to combat depression, as well as to aid in weight loss by helping to regulate appetite.

Two members of the B vitamin family—niacin and inositol—play an important role in helping us sleep. Like other members of the B family, these vitamins help reduce anxiety, which can keep us awake at night. Niacin also aids sleep through its role in synthesizing serotonin. Inositol also helps regulate this important neurotransmitter.

There are a number of herbs on the market that can safely be used to improve sleep quality through a mild sedative effect. These include valerian root, passionflower, hops, lemon balm, chamomile, and skullcap.

Metabolic Booster 6: Sauna

This may seem like an odd component of the metabolic boosters, but taking a sauna will boost your metabolic rate. That's right. You can actually burn extra calories by kicking back with a good book or simply relaxing in the heat. Here's how it works.

Sweating and Calories

You know from experience that when your body heats up, it attempts to cool off by sweating. The heat that causes perspiration can be generated internally from exercise and other activity, or it can be stimulated by an external heat source, like the sun or a sauna. The evaporation of sweat causes a loss of heat from the body.

As our skin becomes wet with sweat, heat is transferred to the liquid on the surface. And when the sweat is sufficiently heated, it vaporizes (turns to gas). As it moves off the skin and into the air, it takes with it heat from the surface of the skin and in the process cools the body. The body uses 0.568 calorie to evaporate 1 gram of sweat. This means that the more you sweat, the more calories you will burn. This is limited only by the speed at which sweat can evaporate. The sweat is produced from lymph fluid, and as this lymph fluid is cycled out of the body, toxins are eliminated.

Saunas

For people who cannot or will not exercise, or as a boost for those who do exercise, saunas are perfect. Not only do saunas cause you to sweat, but the heat they produce also has the effect of raising your metabolic rate, which will make you burn more calories as well. As the body heats up, it cools itself by sending blood from the internal organs to the extremities and closer to the surface of the skin. This in turn heats the skin, and that heat is then transferred out and off of the body when it evaporates as sweat. This whole process increases heart rate, cardiac output, and metabolic rate, much as exercise does. Does this mean that you should use a sauna instead of exercise? Absolutely not, because you don't get the benefits associated with increasing your heart rate and strengthening your muscles. But it's a great way to enhance your metabolic program.

The most popular saunas are classed as either radiant or radiant/far-infrared. Radiant saunas are usually wood or tile boxes or rooms with rocks that can be heated with hot water or electricity. This type of sauna works indirectly. It heats the air, the air then heats the person, and it requires temperatures between 160 and 180 degrees Fahrenheit to induce profuse sweating. This hot air is harsh on a person's skin, and lungs, and requires getting in and out frequently to achieve the cardiovascular and sweating benefits without getting overheated, which can cause headaches or more serious problems.

The radiant/far-infrared sauna uses a white hardwood room and an electric current to heat rods or panels, which then emit far-infrared invisible rays of energy which have wavelengths that are absorbed deeper into the body. These far-infrared rays (FIR) do not heat the air, but are *directly* absorbed by the person in the sauna. This causes the person to perspire profusely with the temperature between 100 and 140 degrees Fahrenheit. Far-infrared is used in hospitals to warm premature infants in incubators, is naturally produced by the sun, and yet strong and effective enough to help relieve pain and stiffness, rid the body of toxins, and provide a safe cardiovascular workout.

In fact, both types of sauna tend to simulate exercise with an increase in pulse rate and cardiac output and with profuse sweating. The result is an increase in overall metabolic activity, with toxins being moved out of the body through sweat and excretion via the liver, kidneys, and intestinal tract. In addition, the sauna increases production of arterial nitric oxide synthetase (NOS) in the same manner that occurs with exercise. NOS is an enzyme that converts arginine into nitric oxide in the arteries. This promotes improved blood flow throughout the vascular system. Sauna therapy has recently been shown to be helpful in treating congestive heart failure.

It is important to gradually increase your time in a sauna and drink enough water to keep up with the sweating. A simple guideline is to consume enough water that you will need to use the bathroom when you get out of the sauna. Staying in the sauna (especially the FIR) for 30 minutes to one hour several times a week can be very beneficial in a weight management program. There are now portable far-infrared saunas available. Portable units are much more affordable and user-friendly for individual use.

Metabolic Booster 7: Detox

As we have seen, there are many factors that play a role in weight loss and weight management. Clinical studies are beginning to demonstrate that chemical toxins are one of these factors.

Various studies have shown that toxins slow down the body's metabolic rate; decrease satiety, resulting in increased caloric intake; and limit your ability to burn fat. The result is that toxins not only can lead to weight gain but can also significantly reduce your ability to lose weight.

I have dedicated an entire chapter to the effects of toxins on weight gain and weight loss (Chapter 9). In that chapter you will learn about these effects and the methods of detoxification.

Chapter 7 Summary

The Fiber35 Diet Metabolic Boosters

- **The Fiber35 Diet Metabolic Formula has seven components:**

    Frequent eating

    Muscle boosting

    Aerobic exercise

    Water, water, water

    Eight hours of sleep

    Sauna

    Detox

- **Each component is very important to maximizing the amount of weight you lose, avoiding the dreaded yo-yo effect, and maintaining your optimum weight for life.**

CHAPTER 8

THE FIBER35 DIET STRENGTH AND CARDIO TRAINING PROGRAM

When you think about strength training, you think of heavy, bulky weights, right? You picture clunky barbells and Mr. Universe. Well, that's the traditional approach. But there's an appealing alternative that offers all the same benefits as well as several unique advantages. It involves the use of tubing and the stretching of flexible elastic bands, which provide a progressive stimulus to your muscles to help build lean mass and increase strength. This approach, used initially in rehabilitation settings, is rapidly becoming the rage in a variety of fitness and sports settings. I personally use the bands in my daily exercise routine, and find that they accommodate my busy lifestyle perfectly, allowing me to work out while traveling without having to look for a gymnasium or load my luggage down with heavy weights. Also, unlike some other forms of exercise, working out with the bands does not aggravate my chronic neck problems. People with pain issues can work safely and comfortably with resistance bands in a number of effective ways.

In this chapter, I'll share with you my simple twenty-minute resistance band protocol, consisting of twenty-six different exercises you can do anytime, anywhere. I'll also offer a longer forty-minute version for those of you who want to maximize the benefits of this simple and exciting approach to strength training. You'll find a list of sources for purchasing your bands in the Resource Directory. For additional information about the Fiber 35 Diet Strength and Cardio training program, visit www.fiber35diet.com.

BEFORE YOU BEGIN

Commencing an exercise program is exciting, and I can't express into words how many benefits await you once you've gotten your body moving and on to a higher level of fitness. But I must also share a few words of caution. All too often I see people jump suddenly into rigorous workouts that leave them tired, strained, and sometimes injured. Before long, they are physically burned out due to muscle fatigue and pure exhaustion, and they lose the motivation to keep going. That's when they stop, and a few months down the road, look back and wonder what went wrong.

Practicing an exercise program shouldn't be like this. You must achieve a fine balance between pushing your body physically, and listening to what it needs (or doesn't need) as you continue forward. If you haven't worked out in a while, I strongly recommend speaking with your physician first. He or she can help you gauge your fitness level so you don't overwork yourself and wind up increasing your risk for injury or illness. You may also have physical limitations that you must consider and with which your doctor can assist you. Exercise should be fun, something that you look forward to every day.

One question I hear frequently is this: When is the best time to exercise? To that I say, "Whenever you can." Everyone's life is busy these days and we all maintain different schedules. For some, it's nearly impossible to get up earlier in the morning to fit in a workout; for others, if the exercise isn't done before 8 a.m., it won't happen at all that day. From a physiological standpoint, there's no definitive answer on the exact time of day that's ideal. There are arguments for both sides—morning and afternoon workouts—and for various reasons. Add to that the fact everyone's body is different, too. Exercise can stimulate one person to feel awake for hours, while it doesn't have such a strong effect on someone else. The biggest challenge for most people is just fitting exercise in at all, no matter what time of day. I recommend experimenting with different times to see how you feel and what fits your personal schedule best. Go with what works for you, simple as that. Aim to schedule your workouts in before your meals, however, so your body can digest properly. If you choose to work out after a meal, try to wait at least two hours, especially if you want to engage in some intense cardio and you've eaten a full meal.

Also, keep in mind that the benefits of exercise are cumulative. So you don't have to spend a full hour in one session. You can split up the time devoted to working out through your day. A little here, a little there. It all adds up!

What to Wear

Get yourself some comfortable workout clothes. Luckily, we have numerous options these days for exercise apparel, or what the retailers like to call activewear. I love the fabrics that help wick away sweat from the skin and keep one dry and comfortable. But you can easily start with just a plain old T-shirt and shorts, and then venture into a store to check out other options. Aside from stand-alone stores that specialize in activewear, most department stores have whole sections devoted to this type of clothing. For women, I suggest investing in a sports bra that provides added support. Wear comfortable shoes, too. Classic sneakers or running shoes are a good choice. Avoid anything with hard soles. You want shoes that are flexible and will allow you to move with ease and comfort.

RESISTANCE BANDS

Unlike exercise machines and dumbbells, bands don't rely on the force of gravity to provide resistance. It's the stretching of the band that creates the resistance: the farther you stretch it, the greater the resistance. It's that simple!

A single band can be used to perform a multitude of exercises that will strengthen every major muscle group in your body. It can even work on some muscles, such as the rotator cuff over the shoulder joint, that machines don't affect. The bands don't just increase strength—they help build flexibility, power, balance, and speed. The result is that these simple, lightweight, inexpensive rubber resistance bands can help you burn off fat while increasing lean muscle mass and improving your overall fitness.

The Advantages of Strength Training and Resistance Bands

Regardless of whether you use bands or elect a more traditional approach to strength training, you can expect to experience a number of benefits, including:

- **Injury prevention through correction of muscle imbalances.**

- **Delay (or even reversal) of muscle mass loss experienced with aging.**

- **Decrease in total cholesterol and improvement in the ratio of good to bad cholesterol (lowering the risk of heart disease).**

- **Increased bone density.**

The use of resistance bands offers all of these benefits, plus:

- **Portability**

- **Low cost**

- **Freedom of motion**

The portability of the bands is based on the fact that they weigh only a few ounces and don't take up much space, fitting easily into your overnight bag or purse. You can go through a complete workout program using just a couple of bands with different resistances. You can also recruit ordinary household items like broom handles, small chairs, and stools to enhance the effect. And you don't need a lot of space to do your routine.

With the aid of resistance bands, your home becomes your gym, without the need for any major modifications or additions to the contents. And the cost of setting up such a tubing gym is amazingly low: under $75. Actually you can get by on much less, because you can get a lot of mileage out of a single band, with an investment of less than $5!

The freedom of motion offered by these bands is inherent in the fact they can be adjusted to accommodate body size and shape and used in virtually any position. With the aid of resistance bands, you can exercise all muscle groups, including the smaller ones. By strengthening these, you help prevent injury.

Basic Terms

Before getting into the specifics of my resistance band workout, I want to familiarize you with some basic terms and concepts, beginning with *repetitions* and *sets*. A repetition (or *rep*) is simply the number of times you perform a given movement. When you perform several repetitions of the same movement in a row, you are doing a set. The basic (twenty-minute) band routine will involve one set of fifteen to twenty reps for each of the band exercises.

The number of sets and reps helps determine the intensity—or amount of stress—on a muscle. The length of time you rest between sets will also influence the intensity. The primary factor influencing intensity, however, is the resistance of the tubing. This is very much a subjective measurement, varying between individuals.

One last term you'll need to know is *recovery*. Your recovery period is the amount of time between workouts that involve the same grouping of muscles. For our purposes, we'll split the body into two muscle groups: upper and lower body. If you do a full workout, involving both these muscle groups, you'll want to skip at least one day between workouts. This translates into working out on three nonconsecutive days per week. Another option is to devote one day to one set of muscles, and then do a workout involving the other set the next day. For example, you may want to do the upper body on Monday and Wednesday and the lower body on Tuesday and Thursday. In this case you may extend the number of sets to fill the time—or keep it constant if you're pressed for time. The important thing to remember is *not* to work any one muscle grouping on consecutive days: always skip a day after you do the full-body workout.

Adjusting Your Bands

The thickness of the band determines the amount of resistance. Intensity of an exercise session increases with the thickness of the bands. So by varying thickness, you can control the amount of resistance, thus tailoring a program to your individual needs. Generally speaking, you'll want to start with thinner bands and progress to thicker ones as you build strength. Some exercises will call for more resistance than others, and thus prompt you to change bands. A good starter set of resistance bands might consist of two or three different sizes.

Have Band, Will Travel

One important consideration in setting up to work with your bands—especially when you travel—is that one end of a band must be anchored to something solid in order for the band to be effectively and safely used. Any solid object will do. This might be a tree if you're outside or a door if you're inside. I recommend a "door anchor." This is strip of heavy-duty nylon webbing that is doubled over to form a loop and placed in the hinge, side, or top of a door. Once the door is closed, the door anchor is wedged solidly in position, and you can simply thread your elastic band through it to hold it securely in place. Once you've invested in a band and a door anchor, you're in business. As long as there's a door nearby, you know you'll be able to set up your "gym"!

Stretching and Cooling Down

Once upon a time stretching was routinely done before exercise, as a warmup. That is no longer the case. Experts now agree that stretching should be done only after a muscle has been worked. This is because once a muscle has been used, it will be easier to stretch, since it now has a higher core temperature and thus a greater blood flow. By stretching a fatigued muscle, you prevent tightening, increase flexibility, and help it recover faster. You'll get maximal benefit out of each stretch by holding it for thirty to sixty seconds.

You may want to incorporate stretching with the cooldown period following your workout session. This is when your body functions are stabilizing—your previously elevated heart rate is normalizing and you stop perspiring. During this period, you'll want to drink some water and relax in a quiet environment, while gently stretching your fatigued muscles, one group at a time.

Caution: If any of these exercises cause pain or are uncomfortable for you, do not do them. Always check with your physician before starting an exercise program. You can easily take this routine to your doctor to get his or her approval.

THE WORKOUT

My upper body workout involves three exercises for the back and chest, four for the shoulders, two for the biceps, and three for the triceps. These exercises and the primary muscles they recruit are listed below.

Exercises and the Muscles They Involve: Upper Body

Back

Lat Pull-Down	Latissimus dorsi
Low Row	Teres major
Stiff Arm Pull-Down	Trapezius, Rhomboideus major, Posterior deltoids, Triceps brachii

Chest

Push-Ups	Pectoralis major
Chest Press	Anterior deltoid
Flys	Tricep brachii

Shoulders

Shoulder Press	Anterior, middle, and posterior deltoids
Side Lateral	Teres major and minor
Shrugs (optional)	Trapezius
Reverse Fly	Infraspinatas, Rhomboideus

Exercises and the Muscles They Involve: Upper Body (continued)

Biceps

Bi Curl	Brachialis
Alternate Bi Curl	Biceps brachii

Triceps

Triceps Push-Down	Medial tricep
Overhead Triceps Extension	Long tricep
Kickback	Lateral head tricep

My lower body workout involves eight exercises designed to work the muscles of the legs and three to work the abdominal muscles as indicated below.

Exercises and the Muscles They Involve: Lower Body

Legs

Squat	Rectus femoris, Vastus lateralis, Vastus intermedius, Gluteus medius, Gluteus maximus
Stationary Lunge	Rectus femoris, Vastus lateralis, Vastus intermedius, Gluteus maximus
Wide Squat	Vastus lateralis, Rectus femoris, Vastus medialis, Adductor, Gracilis, Gluteus maximus
Dead Lift	Semitendinosus, Bifemoris, Semimembranosus, Gluteus maximus
Outer Thigh Hip Abduction	Gluteus medius, Gluteus maximus, Tensor facia latae
Floor Hip Extension	Gluteus maximus, Biceps femoris
Inner Thigh Adduction	Adductor longus, Adductor magnus, Gracilis pectineus
Calf Raise	Gastrocnemius, Medial head, Lateral head, Soleus

Exercises and the Muscles They Involve: Lower Body (continued)

Abdominals	
Overhead Crunches	Rectus abdominis, Oblique
Wood Chops	Rectus abdominis
Side Bends	Oblique

If you choose to work both upper and lower body at the same session, you'll want to do either one set of each of the above exercises (fifteen to twenty reps each), for a total workout period of twenty minutes; or two sets of each, for a total workout period of forty minutes. Make sure to take at least one day off between workouts, but do at least three workouts per week. If you wish to work out more often, then alternate your upper body workouts with your lower body workouts. If you do this, you can safely work out on a daily basis should you choose to do so. Three times per week is sufficient, however.

UPPER BODY PROGRAM

For Your Back

Lat Pull-Down

Anchor the middle of your band to the top of a door. Facing the anchor, either kneel on the ground or stand, and grasp both handles of the band, using an overhand grip, with palms facing the floor. Hands should be just slightly wider apart than shoulder width, with arms extended out in front of you (not over your head). Lean backward slightly (about 10 degrees), and pull the band back and toward each side of your chest. Exhale as you pull down. Reverse your movement slowly as you inhale, keeping your body still. Repeat fifteen to twenty times in succession. If you are doing two sets, rest for no more than thirty seconds between sets.

Low Row

Anchor your band to a door at waist level. Facing the door, grasp both ends of the band with an overhand grip, with palms facing each other. Take a few steps backward, so that the band is taut. Bend knees slightly, straighten back, tighten abdominal muscles, and pull band toward you with both hands as far as you can, keeping arms tight to sides. Exhale as you do this; inhale as you return the band to its original position. Repeat fifteen to twenty times in succession. If you are doing two sets, rest for no more than thirty seconds between sets.

Stiff Arm Pull-Down

Anchor your band to the top of a door. Stand at arm's length from the door, with arms extended out in front of you. Grasp the ends of the band with an overhand grip, hands placed slightly wider than shoulder width apart. Exhale and keep your arms straight as you pull both ends of the band down, stopping at your hips. Inhale as you return the band to its original position. Repeat fifteen to twenty times in succession. If you are doing two sets, rest for no more than thirty seconds between sets.

For Your Chest

Push-Ups

Assume the traditional push-up position on the floor: palms of hands flat on floor slightly more than shoulder width apart; legs straight, with weight on balls of the feet; feet just a few inches apart. If you find this exercise too difficult, you may modify the basic position by having your knees, rather than the balls of your feet, touch the floor. Inhale as you lower your body to the floor; exhale as you lift it. Repeat fifteen to twenty times in succession. If you are doing two sets, rest for no more than thirty seconds between sets. Note: No bands are used with this exercise.

Chest Press

Anchor your band to a door at chest height. Standing with your feet shoulder width apart and one foot slightly in front of the other, face away from the door, holding one end of the band in each hand. Thrust your arms forward, extending them full length, as you exhale. Inhale as you return arms to their original position. Repeat fifteen to twenty times in succession. If you are doing two sets, rest for no more than thirty seconds between sets.

Flys

Anchor band in side of door about shoulder height. Stand with one foot in front of the other, facing away from the door. Grasping one end of the band in each hand with an overhand grip, bend forward about 30 degrees. Bend elbows slightly while pulling the handles together in front of you, making a circular motion. Exhale as you make this motion; inhale as you return your arms to their original position. Repeat fifteen to twenty times in succession. If you are doing two sets, rest for no more than thirty seconds between sets.

For Your Shoulders

Shoulder Press

Stand on the middle of a band, holding one end in each hand at the level of your waist. Grasp the handles in an overhand grip, lifting to shoulder height, while exhaling. Palms will be facing away from your body; feet will be shoulder width apart, and back will be just slightly arched. Now lift the ends of the band above your head, extending your arms completely, while continuing to exhale. Inhale as you bend your elbows and return the band to its original position. Repeat fifteen to twenty times in succession. If you are doing two sets, rest for no more than thirty seconds between sets.

Side Laterals

Stand on the middle of a band, holding one end in each hand at the level of your waist. Have your palms facing each other as you grasp the handles. With elbows slightly bent, lift arms to your sides as you exhale, stopping at shoulder level when they are parallel to the ground. Pause, and then inhale as you slowly lower your arms to their original position. Repeat fifteen to twenty times in succession. If you are doing two sets, rest for no more than thirty seconds between sets.

Shrugs (Optional)

With feet shoulder width apart and knees slightly bent, stand on the middle of a band, holding one end in each hand (overhand grip) at hip level, with your palms facing your legs. Now raise your shoulders (shrug them) as high as possible toward the back of your ears as you exhale. Pause momentarily, and then slowly return shoulders to their original position as you inhale. Repeat fifteen to twenty times in succession. If you are doing two sets, rest for no more than thirty seconds between sets.

Reverse Fly

Anchor the middle of your band in the door at shoulder level, facing the door. Placing one leg slightly in front of the other, grasp the handles. Keeping elbows slightly bent, pull the band outward and back, as you exhale. Inhale as you return the band to its original position. Repeat fifteen to twenty times in succession. If you are doing two sets, rest for no more than thirty seconds between sets.

For Your Biceps

Bi Curl

Stand on the middle of a band, grasping handles with an underhand grip. Begin with your hands at hip level, palms up and elbows to your sides. Exhale while curling the ends of the band inward toward your body. Inhale as you return your hands to their original position. Repeat fifteen to twenty times in succession. If you are doing two sets, rest for no more than thirty seconds between sets. Note: By moving your feet further apart, you will increase the tension on the band, thus increasing the difficulty of the exercise.

Alternate Bi Curl

Stand on the middle of a band, grasping handles with an underhand grip. Begin with your hands at hip level, palms up and elbows to your sides. Exhale while curling the end of *one* band inward toward your body. Inhale as you return that hand to its original position. Repeat the same motion with the other hand. As you lower one hand, start to raise the other. Repeat fifteen to twenty times in succession. If you are doing two sets, rest for no more than thirty seconds between sets. Note: By moving your feet farther apart, you will increase the tension on the band, thus increasing the difficulty of the exercise.

For Your Triceps

Triceps Push-Down

Anchor the middle of your band to the top of a door. Grasp the handles, keeping elbows bent and to your sides. Exhale as you straighten your arms to your sides. Pause momentarily. Inhale. Bring your bands back to starting position (chest height). Repeat fifteen to twenty times in succession. If you are doing two sets, rest for no more than thirty seconds between sets.

Overhead Triceps Extension

Stand with one foot on middle of band. Grasp handles. Put other foot forward through band. Bring hands behind head, elbows pointing toward the ceiling. Straighten arms as you reach up. Exhale and repeat. Repeat fifteen to twenty times in succession. If you are doing two sets, rest for no more than thirty seconds between sets.

Kickback

Anchor band to door at waist level. Grasp handles with overhand grip, arms against sides and elbows bent 90 degrees. Bend at waist, with knees slightly bent. Keeping arms close to your sides and parallel to the ground. Straighten them out as you exhale. Reverse the movement slowly while inhaling. Repeat fifteen to twenty times in succession. If you are doing two sets, rest for no more than thirty seconds between sets.

LOWER BODY PROGRAM

For Your Legs

Squat

Stand on the middle of a band with feet shoulder width apart, grasping one end of the band in each hand. Elevate handles to shoulder length, holding them just to the sides of your shoulders. Stand straight with your head erect, chest out, and shoulders back. You want your back to be slightly arched at the base and your toes to be pointed outward at a 30- to 35-degree angle. You'll inhale while lowering your buttocks toward the floor, simultaneously tightening your torso muscles. Stop when the tops of your thighs are parallel to the floor. Keep your head up and torso muscles tight as you lift back up to a standing position while inhaling. Exhale as you come up; inhale as you come down. Repeat fifteen to twenty times in succession. If you are doing two sets, rest for no more than thirty seconds between sets.

Stationary Lunge

Stand on the middle of a band. Grasping one end of the band in each hand, raise your hands to shoulder height. Step backward with one leg, bending the front leg to 90 degrees. The rear leg should also be bent slightly. While keeping your torso upright, push off the heel of your front foot and straighten your front leg. Now lower yourself back to your original position. Repeat fifteen to twenty times in succession. Then return to the upright position. Switch legs and repeat for the same number of reps. If you are doing two sets, rest for no more than thirty seconds between sets.

Wide Squat

Stand on a band with legs wide apart and toes pointed out. Pick up handles. Breathe in while lowering your torso until the tops of your thighs are parallel to the ground. Keep your back flat and buttocks back. Exhale and stand. Repeat. Keep tension on band. Repeat fifteen to twenty times in succession. If you are doing two sets, rest for no more than thirty seconds between sets.

Dead Lift

Stand with both feet on band, with feet hip width apart. Grasp handles with overhand grip, palms facing body, holding bands close to your shins. Bend forward at the hip, with knees bent slightly (about 10 degrees). Keep your back nearly flat, head up, chest out, and shoulders back. Holding the band as close as possible to your body, slowly stand straight while keeping your arms bent and your back flat. Exhale as you do this. Keep torso muscles contracted, tightening your buttocks as you straighten up and inhale. Reverse your movements, slowly lowering handles back to starting position. Repeat fifteen to twenty times in succession. If you are doing two sets, rest for no more than thirty seconds between sets.

Outer Thigh Hip Abduction

Attach band to a door at ankle height. Face sideways and put one foot through the handle. Stand tall with feet shoulder width apart. Hold onto a nearby solid object for support. Now as you maintain your upright stance, exhale and move the leg with the band sideways as far as you can. Pause and return to original position as you inhale. Repeat fifteen to twenty times in succession. Then do the same with the other leg. If you are doing two sets, rest for no more than thirty seconds between sets.

Floor Hip Extension

Kneel on your hands and knees while holding one end of a band under your right hand. Put your right foot into the handle of the band, so that the ball of that foot rests against the handle. Lift that leg, and stretch it straight out so that it is just above and parallel to the floor. Exhale as you do this. Now, as you inhale, bring your knee as close to your chest as you can. Repeat fifteen to twenty times, and then do the same with the opposite leg. If you are doing two sets, rest for no more than thirty seconds between sets.

Inner Thigh Adduction

Anchor band to a door at ankle height. Face sideways and put one foot through the handle. Stand tall with feet shoulder width apart. Hold onto a nearby solid object for support. Extend working leg 18 to 24 inches to the side of your body. Move that leg across your body as far as you can, while maintaining an upright stance and exhaling. Return slowly to your original position as you inhale. Avoid bending at the waist. Repeat fifteen to twenty times in succession. Change legs and do the same. If you are doing two sets, rest for no more than thirty seconds between sets.

Calf Raise

Stand with your feet shoulder width apart on top of a band. Raise the handles of that band just above your shoulders behind your head. Now rise up on your toes as high as you can, while exhaling. Pause momentarily before inhaling as you lower your heels to the floor. Keep your legs straight throughout this exercise, but do not lock them. Repeat fifteen to twenty times in succession. If you are doing two sets, rest for no more than thirty seconds between sets.

For Your Abdomen

Overhead Crunches

Anchor a band to the top of a door and kneel directly in front of it, facing in the opposite direction, while grasping the handle with both hands. As you exhale, pull the handle down until your hands are level with the top of your head. Now bend down until your elbows make contact with your knees. Return to your original position as you inhale. Repeat fifteen to twenty times in succession. If you are doing two sets, rest for no more than thirty seconds between sets.

Wood Chops

Secure a band over the top of a door. Take a step back so that tension is on the band. Standing directly in front of it, grasp the handle with both hands. Keep your arms straight, and pull the band down as you exhale, bending at the waist as if you were chopping wood. Repeat fifteen to twenty times in succession. If you are doing two sets, rest for no more than thirty seconds between sets.

Side Bends

Stand on the middle of a band, with handles at your side, band stretched tightly. Feet should be shoulder width apart. Lean to one side slowly as you exhale, and run your hand down the side of your leg as far as you comfortably can. The other arm will be simultaneously pulling up the other side of the band. Keep that arm against the side of your body. Inhale as you return to your original upright position, and lean to the other side in the same manner. Keep your hands against the sides of your body throughout the entire exercise to make sure you're bending properly. Repeat fifteen to twenty times in succession. If you are doing two sets, rest for no more than thirty seconds between sets.

DON'T FORGET YOUR CARDIO!

Now that you've nailed down your resistance band regimen, it's time to incorporate cardiovascular exercise. Exactly which cardio exercises you do and how often you do them is very much a matter of personal choice. I probably do more cardio than most people because I find it extremely benefecial and enjoyable; but it's not necessary to do more than three thirty-minute cardiovascular workout sessions per week to reap the benefits of these powerful and invigorating activities.

If you've elected to do the full-body resistance band program in a single session, I recommend that you simply add a cardio exercise on alternate days. That can be walking either on the ground or on a treadmill (or any aerobic-type sport, such as swimming). If you're unaccustomed to any type of physical activity, you'll want to start with walking at a normal pace, gradually increasing your speed. (Don't forget to inhale and exhale deeply as you move!) If you're already a seasoned walker, just keep on doing what you're doing, or join the world of power walking if you're so moved. The type of cardio exercise or activity you do is not nearly as important as how you do it, how often you do it, and how long you do it. As to the first of these concerns, just keep in mind that cardio is all about increasing the workload of your lungs and heart. Leisurely, slow-paced strolls won't do this, though they're a good place to start.

If you're already working out six days a week, doing upper body and lower body resistance band routines on alternate days, just add a thirty-minute cardio session on three of those days. The charts below show two optional exercise schedules. Use these—or create your own schedule as long as it includes full-body resistance band training three times per week and thirty minutes of cardio three times weekly.

Schedule 1

Monday	Tuesday	Wednesday	Thursday	Friday	Saturday	Sunday
bands: full-body 20–40 minutes	walk 30 minutes	bands: full-body 20–40 minutes	walk 30 minutes	bands: full-body 20–40 minutes	walk 30 minutes	rest

Schedule 2

Monday	Tuesday	Wednesday	Thursday	Friday	Saturday	Sunday
bands: upper 20 minutes	bands: lower 20 minutes	bands: upper 20 minutes	bands: lower 20 minutes	rest	bands: upper 20 minutes	bands: lower 20 minutes
walk 30 minutes	walk or rest	walk 30 minutes	walk 30 minutes	rest	walk 30 minutes	walk or rest

The one day of rest is optional but recommended.

CHAPTER 9

THE FIBER35 DIET DETOXIFICATION FACTOR

Weight management isn't confined to a cookie-cutter list of things to do (or not do). If that were the case, then we'd all simply check off each item and be on our merry, skinny way. Unfortunately, many factors play a role in weight management, and science continues to uncover new mysteries with regard to weight loss.

Up to now, we have seen that in order to lose weight you must manage the primary factors, including lowering your caloric intake; increasing your metabolism; and eating the proper mix and type of proteins, carbohydrates, fats, and, of course, fiber. We also know that the success of these weight loss strategies varies considerably from one individual to another. So other factors come in to play that need our attention. Chief among these are the chemical toxins that infiltrate our daily lives. Clinical studies are beginning to demonstrate their profound effect on our health and our ability to stay lean.

Various studies have shown that toxins slow down the body's metabolic rate; decrease feelings of fullness, leading to eating more and more calories; and limit our ability to burn fat. Toxins can not only lead to weight gain but also sabotage your ability to lose weight.

WHAT ARE TOXINS?

Today the term *toxin* is used to described anything that is foreign or poisonous to the body. Although we can certainly have toxic relatives, toxic thoughts, or toxic relationships, I generally use the term *toxic* in discussing two broad classes of toxins: environmental and internal. Environmental toxins include household chemicals, industrial pollutants, food additives, and pesticides. Internal toxins consist of waste products created by normal metabolic processes within the body. Such digestive toxins are produced as a result of breaking down proteins, starches, and fats.

Environmental Toxins

Since the industrial revolution, we have lived with the concept of environmental toxins. Over the last 100 years we have introduced at least 75,000 new chemicals into our environment.[1] For most of these, there have been no long-term studies proving that they are safe for human consumption or exposure. In fact, most of them are known to be unsafe for humans at some level.

Among of the most frequently studied types of environmental toxins are the organochlorines (OCs). These were widely used industrial toxins and were found in insecticides, plastics, and industrial oils. One of the best-known OCs is DDT, which has been banned from use in the United States because of its toxicity but still remains in our environment. The reason OCs get so much attention is that they are stored in fat cells for long periods of time. One particular study stated, "OCs are found in virtually every person on the planet."[2] Numerous other studies support the idea that we are living in a world full of toxins.

In a large collaborative study organized by the Mount Sinai School of Medicine in New York, scientists found an average of ninety-one industrial compounds, pollutants, and other toxic chemicals in the blood and urine of nine volunteer test subjects. These volunteers were tested for toxins precisely because they were in normal health and were not employed in occupations that exposed them to industrial chemicals. None lived in an area polluted by nearby industrial facilities.

Despite an apparently uncontaminated lifestyle, every single person in this study tested positive for seventy-seven toxic chemicals or more. (These toxins found in the body are called a person's "body burden."[3]) Of the 167 chemicals isolated from the bodily fluids of this test group, seventy-six are known to cause cancer in humans or animals, ninety-four are toxic to brain tissue and the nervous system, and seventy-nine can cause birth defects or abnormal development. What is particularly disturbing about this test is that it probably underestimates the total toxic level in the body, because the researchers tested only blood and urine. We know that the body stores toxins in fat cells, so the total body burden is very likely higher than urine and blood tests would demonstrate.

Further support for the uncomfortable idea that we live in an increasingly toxic world comes from the U.S. government's Centers for Disease Control and Prevention (CDC). In a National Report on Human Exposure to Environmental Chemicals, the CDC found that of 116 environmental toxins used in consumer products or released in industrial pollution, eighty-nine showed up in tests of people's blood and urine. According to the report, PCBs, dioxins, phthalates, organophosphate pesticides, herbicides, pest repellants, and disinfectants were among the chemical toxins revealed in lab analyses.[4] These tests found that toxins were present in significant numbers in virtually every person tested.

Hence, the notion that we live in a toxic world is very true.

TOXINS CAUSE WATER AND FAT RETENTION
When faced with toxicity, our bodies respond by retaining water, in an effort to dilute water-soluble toxins; and fat, to try to dilute fat-soluble toxins. Your body will store water and fat in an effort to dilute these toxins.

Internal Toxins

It's more difficult to understand the concept of internal toxicity. Everyday physiological processes such as energy production, digestion, and hormone synthesis create waste products that, if not discarded, interfere with the function of our internal organs. Internal toxicity is the process by which the body produces destructive toxic substances. As humans we perform only two broad physiological functions. First, we take in and absorb nutrients. Second, we expel toxins. We excrete these toxins mostly when we urinate (release urine) or eliminate (release fecal matter), but also to a lesser degree when we breathe, sweat, cut our hair, and trim our nails.

Most of these wastes are by-products of the air we breathe and the food we eat. However, our intestinal tracts are full of bacteria and yeast that also produce waste. These bacteria and yeast are often called gut flora or intestinal microbes. Some of these bacteria are highly beneficial. They assist in the digestion of some vitamins, and they play a significant role in our immune response. About 100 trillion (3 pounds) of these bacteria live in the intestinal tract of virtually every human on earth. In fact, we have more of these microbes living in our intestinal tract than we have cells in our body (there are only about 80 trillion cells). These bacteria are either good for you, bad for you, or neutral.

The good bacteria are often called probiotics (a term that means "for life") because of the role they play in keeping us healthy. These good bacteria produce substances like lactic and acetic acid, which help to destroy harmful bacteria. Two examples of these good bacteria are *Lactobacillus acidophilus* and *Bifidobacteria bifidum*.

We also have bad intestinal flora. Some examples of bad flora are salmonella and *Candida albicans,* a yeast that can cause an infection when it grows out of control. This is the same yeast that causes some women to get vaginal yeast infections. These bad flora are constantly taking in nutrients and creating wastes in the form of indol, skatol, and methane, to name a few.[5] Methane is an internally produced toxin that results in gas and bloating. Long-term production of these internal toxins can lead to a weakened immune system, inflammation, and a slower metabolic rate.

Toxins Can Be Passed on to Our Children

As medical researchers learn more about toxins, there is a growing consensus that toxins play a central role in damaging our health. They take a toll from the time you are in your mother's womb until your last breath. What's more, they may even harm you before you are conceived.

In laboratory tests at Washington State University, scientists found that fungicides and pesticides used in the United States don't affect just those who are alive and exposed to the direct source. They can change a person's genetics, which then get passed on through many generations.[6] It's remarkable to think that environmental toxins can permanently reprogram inherited traits, altering our evolutionary biology, but the scientific proof is finally emerging. In other words, your great grandparents' genetic legacy, eventually handed down to you, may have been damaged by toxins. And toxins that you are exposed to may cause damage in your great-grandchildren!

TOXINS AND OBESITY

We discussed earlier a group of toxins called organochlorines (OCs). Because they are found in virtually everyone and are easy to detect and measure, OCs are frequently studied in association with obesity.[7] We cannot get rid of them very well, so the body stores them in our fat cells. The more fat you have, the more toxins you retain. As we lose weight, the fat cells release the toxins into the bloodstream. Once these toxins are in the bloodstream, they can cause all kinds of trouble. Detoxification is the process of binding up these toxins and releasing them from the body.

Although the study of detoxification and its impact on obesity is relatively new, we do understand some of the mechanisms of how toxins affect weight gain. In particular, toxins can affect your ability to achieve your weight loss goals in three important ways:

- **Toxins slow down your metabolism.**

- **Toxins decrease your ability to burn fat.**

- **Toxins slow down the time it takes for you to feel full (this is called the satiety response time).**

If you're having a hard time losing weight, it may be a result of the toxins getting dumped into your bloodstream as the fat burns off.

Toxins Slow Your Metabolism

In the past it was thought that your resting metabolic rate (RMR) declined with weight loss primarily because of the decrease in caloric intake or changes in the muscle-to-fat ratio. But clinical studies are now showing just how "toxic" internal toxins can be to efforts to lose weight. One of the first things toxins do when your fat cells release them into the blood is slow down your resting metabolic rate. So as you begin to lose weight, those surfacing toxins can begin to work against your weight loss.

One study that came out in 2002 looked at five factors that affected RMR during weight loss in sixteen obese men—all of whom experienced a decrease in their resting metabolic rate. Not only were toxic OCs in their blood partly to blame for the lower RMR, but the study also confirmed that of the five factors considered, including fat mass and appetite hormones, the presence of OCs was the most important factor influencing the dampened resting metabolic rate.[8] The study further determined that the toxins were affecting the production of the thyroid hormones. Your thyroid plays a major role in your body's regulation of its metabolic rate, so it's not surprising that toxins present in the blood can lead to a slower metabolism.

What this means is that if you can eliminate the toxins from the body fast enough during or before weight loss, you may be able to reduce the decline in your metabolism.

Toxins Decrease Your Ability to Burn Fat

The last thing you want to hear is that something floating around in your blood is preventing your body from burning fat. But that's what these toxins can do. And studies going back more than thirty years indicate that such toxins can hinder the efficiency of your fat-burning systems. In a study in 1971, for example, the University of Nevada's Division of Biochemistry determined that chemical toxins weakened by 20 percent a special coenzyme that the body needs to burn fat! In a more recent study, done in 2002, researchers concluded that toxins released during weight loss had the capacity to damage the fat-burning mitochondria.[9] The damage was significant enough to lower the body's ability to burn calories and, in effect, fat.

Toxins Slow Down the Satiety Response

In his book *Ultra-Metabolism,* Mark Hyman, M.D., states that toxins stored in our fat cells can prevent us from receiving signals from the hormone leptin, which, as you'll recall, is involved in feeding behaviors and hunger. He concluded that over time this could affect the receptor sites in the brain that tell us when we are full.[10] The result is that we either overeat (because the signals take too long to register the satiety response) or are constantly hungry. Either way, it's certain that we will consume more calories and have a harder time maintaining the proper weight.

The question then is: what can we do to cleanse and eliminate toxins from our body, and how can that help us achieve our weight loss goals?

WHAT CAN YOU DO ABOUT TOXINS?

No one can live in a bubble that's free of toxins. Let's be realistic. But we must somehow address the cruel reality that we all carry more than 100 chemical pollutants, pesticides, and toxic metals in our bodies.[11] When your weight loss begins to falter, it's time to consider those other variables that aren't so obvious at first—that aren't about calories in or calories out. I have devised a simple two-step program to help you reduce your exposure to toxins and to lose weight.

Step 1: Minimize toxins in your environment.

Eat organic foods.

Use natural cleaners.

Install water and air filters.

Step 2: Remove toxins from your body.

Detoxify and cleanse.

Exercise.

Take saunas.

Try herbal cleansing programs and supplements.

Consider colon hydrotherapy.

Step 1: Minimize Toxins in Your Environment

Limiting the toxins in your environment is easy to recommend, but harder to achieve. Here are some things you can do:

Eat organic fruits and vegetables whenever possible to avoid the chemicals, pesticides, and herbicides generally found in produce.

Choose organic meats to avoid the hormones and antibiotics found in nonorganic meats.

Choose unprocessed foods so as to avoid preservatives, dyes, nitrates, and nitrites.

Choose natural products to clean your home environment. There are many brands on the market that do not contain harsh chemicals but work very well. Also, try to choose skin and hair products that contain minimal chemicals and dyes. As we mentioned, the skin is a source of absorption as well as elimination.

Change the air conditioning filters in your house often. Get the ducts cleaned yearly. Installing a total house water filter can help eliminate the chlorine and other chemicals found in your water. Use plants such as spider, aloe, and philodendrons to help filter your household air.

Step 2: Remove Toxins from Your Body

Getting rid of the toxins already in your body is a little more difficult. We have seen that the body stores toxins in the fat cells. The question is: what can we do to get the toxins out of the fat cells and out of the body? The answer is detoxification and cleansing, which you can do through a variety of options that we'll explore shortly.

Detoxification and cleansing are crucial to good health. In addition to environmental toxins, the very act of living creates poisons that must be transported out of the body. Detoxification and cleansing are the general terms for the collection and elimination of these poisons. In general, detoxification is the collection of toxins and cleansing is the process of eliminating the toxins from the body.

Internal detoxification and cleansing are as old as the idea of health. Four thousand years ago, according to the earliest medical textbook ever discovered (the Ebers Papyrus, found in the sands of Egypt), physicians were already using enemas to help the body cleanse and fight off disease. Around the year 400 BCE, Hippocrates, the Greek doctor generally accepted as the father of western medicine, gave his patients cleansing herbs to help their bodies heal. Galen, a highly influential Greek physician born in 129 CE, believed cleansing was crucial to keeping the body in balance and good health.

In the twentieth century, Dr. Bernard Jensen pioneered many of our current ideas about cleansing. In his book *Dr. Jensen's Guide to Diet and Detoxification: Healthy Secrets from Around the World,* Dr. Jensen warns, "We all need to work toward a fully nourishing, toxin-free food regimen that provides all the right nutrients for building new tissue while promoting adequate elimination of normal wastes and toxins from both internal processes and the external environment."[12]

With that in mind, let's review the most accessible and common ways to detox and cleanse.

Exercise

Exercise is of course one of the most important things you can do for your overall health. Everyone recommends exercise for weight loss because it burns calories and increases your metabolism. As it relates to detoxification, exercise serves several functions. First, exercise moves the lymphatic system. The role of the lymphatic system is to gather toxins. Once gathered, the toxins must be eliminated from the body. Exercise helps out here as well. During exercise the lymphatic system dumps toxins into the circulatory system, where they can be processed by the liver and eliminated through the bladder or colon. Finally, exercise helps you sweat out toxins.

For many people, however, the thought of exercise (espe exercise) is overwhelming. It's important to begin to increase you

If you have not exercised in a while, you should begin with lo or stretching. Go easy until you build up your cardiovascular s contains all my recommendations and instructions for starting a Be patient with yourself as you start an exercise program.

Saunas

Earlier, I covered the benefits of saunas in speeding up your metabolism. Saunas, as well as steam baths and hot bathtub soaks, are also great for sweating out unwanted toxins. Sweating occurs naturally during physical activity, but it can be induced through either a sauna or a bath. Each can be very therapeutic as well, offering a host of health benefits. Because your core body temperature gets raised a little, you actually boost your immune system by disabling or killing microbes and improving circulation. You also further increase your production of growth hormone. In fact, upping your core body temperature is one of the few known ways to stimulate increased production of growth hormone, which helps your body shed fat while maintaining lean muscle mass.

The health benefits of saunas in particular are numerous. The skin is the largest organ of your body, and a prime participant in elimination. Because of its size and area, it actually eliminates more cellular waste, through the pores, than the colon and kidneys combined. It's one of your body's seven channels of detoxification.

SEVEN CHANNELS OF DETOXIFICATION

Among the most powerful methods of routine detoxification and cleaning is relying on your own body's machinery. Your body is equipped with organs and systems responsible for collecting, filtering, and helping eliminate the toxins that perpetually accumulate. Specifically, we all have five organs and two fluids that are involved in detoxification and cleansing. Together they are called the seven channels of detoxification. These are as follows.

1. Lungs—The lungs dispense toxins with every exhalation. Chief among these toxins is carbon dioxide, a by-product of respiration, the body's release of energy. The muscular contractions involved in breathing also help to transport lymph and blood, which also convey toxins. The lungs' lining of mucus and cilia (small hairs that capture airborne particles) helps prevent toxins from entering the body.

2. **Liver**—Health researchers believe that in today's polluted world, the added toxic burden on the liver contributes to chronic fatigue, high cholesterol, irritable bowel syndrome, cognitive difficulties, and high blood pressure. A major organ of elimination, the liver serves as the manager of the entire detoxification process in the body.

3. **Colon**—The colon is the final place in the body where waste (food residue) travels before being eliminated. It is critical that bowel elimination happens daily.

4. **Kidneys**—The kidneys filter out water-soluble wastes from the blood that flows to them from the liver. These wastes are then stored in the bladder before elimination through the urine.

5. **Skin**—As a protective covering, it keeps toxins from entering the body. Simultaneously, because of its size and area, it actually eliminates more cellular waste than the colon and kidneys combined.

6. **Blood**—The blood that moves through the cardiovascular system is a key transportation system in the body, bringing nutrients and oxygen to the cells and flushing away waste products and toxins.

7. **Lymph**—Lymph, a clear fluid filled with immune cells called lymphocytes, moves around the body in a series of vessels that parallel the paths of the veins. Lymph delivers nutrients, collects cellular waste, and helps destroy pathogens.

These channels must work together in harmony for detoxification and cleansing to be maximized.

JUMP-START YOUR WEIGHT LOSS WITH A CLEANSE

As we have discussed, clinical studies have shown that toxins released from the fat cells during weight loss inhibit our ability to lose more, and to maintain our ideal weight. These toxins may, in fact, be the primary reason that our metabolism slows during weight loss. This is why it's critical that our detoxification and cleansing systems are performing at maximum efficiency when we begin a weight loss program.

Because it can be difficult to know whether or not your body's natural detox systems are operating efficiently, I often recommend doing a test through a natural health practitioner that can help you determine this. Several tests are available, one of which is the Comprehensive Detoxification Profile offered by, among others, Genova Diagnostics of North Carolina. (Refer to the Resource Directory for more information.) This test introduces a substance like caffeine or acetaminophen and then uses saliva, urine, and blood samples to measure how well your body naturally detoxifies using its own internal systems. It helps show how efficient your body is at processing foreign substances, and it's usually available through natural health practitioners. Other tests can measure the presence and level of toxins in your body, such as the heavy metals lead, mercury, and arsenic.

I have always been a big fan of using herbs, supplements, and diet to improve the efficiency of the detoxification process. I have seen great successes in my clinics with people who have lost weight and improved their health. On the basis of your level of "toxification," I would suggest a program of herbs, supplements, and food that can help you maximize your weight loss by improving each of the seven channels of detoxification.

Most cleansing and detoxification kits contain two formulas (in two different bottles) in a single box. The first bottle usually is a detoxification formula containing natural herbs that help pull toxins from the organs. The second bottle contains different herbs and minerals that help the colon eliminate the toxins more efficiently. You want to look for an internal cleanse system that is designed as follows.

- **Detox formula: Select an all-natural formula containing a variety of herbs to support the kidneys (parsley), lungs (mullein), skin (oatstraw), lymphatic system (echinacea), blood (blessed thistle), and liver. Liver support is of primary importance and is provided by herbs like burdock root, dandelion leaf and root, turmeric, and yellow dock root. Added liver support is provided by the addition of N-acetyl-cysteine and alpha lipoic acid. Look for a formula containing all these herbs, as well as others (like oregano leaf, fenugreek seed, and garlic bulb) to support the elimination channels. The addition of kelp will also support the elimination process, as well as the endocrine system, especially your thyroid, thus helping to increase your metabolism.**

- **Colon support: This is important enough to merit its own formulation. Look for a formula containing gentle, nonirritating herbs like alder buckthorn, okra, triphala and aloe, and the mineral magnesium hydroxide that will soothe the bowel, stimulate peristalsis, and help eliminate mucus from the bowel.**

You will also want to add extra fiber to your diet during the cleanse because fiber helps absorb and sweep the toxins out of the colon.

Note: These cleanse kits can be found at most health food stores. You can use these kits while on the Fiber35 Diet. They do not require fasting. For more information about where you can find cleansing systems, refer to the Resource Directory.

It's a good idea to jump-start your metabolism before starting an exercise program by following a whole-body detoxification program that will cleanse all channels of elimination. There are many approaches to cleansing and detoxification. Depending on your individual needs and preferences, you will want to choose a fifteen-day or thirty-day cleanse as described below:

Fifteen-Day Cleanse

If you are a first-time cleanser, or if you have not cleansed in the last six months, or if you have daily bowel movements, you'll want to select whole-herb cleanse that gently supports all the channels of elimination. This support is best provided with a two-part formula: (1) an evening formula to encourage mild elimination through the bowel using a variety of herbs (like marshmallow root, rhubarb root, and buckthorn bark) and enzymes; and (2) a morning formula, which contains a synergistic blend of a variety of herbs (mostly liver-supporting) and enzymes to support the remaining organs of elimination. These two-week cleanse programs are great if you plan to stay on Phase One for two weeks.

Thirty-Day Cleanse

If you have completed an internal cleanse before or simply want a longer cleanse, your best choice is a thirty-day total-body cleanse that contains high-potency herbal extracts and whole herbs designed to support the body's seven channels of elimination. Here again, you'll want to look for a two-part formula: (1) an evening formula that contains herbs and magnesium hydroxide to hydrate and enhance elimination through the bowel, and (2) a morning formula that blends a variety of whole herbs with high-potency powdered extracts to support the remaining channels of elimination. These thirty-day cleanse programs are great if you plan to stay on Phase One for a month.

Completing one (or more) of the above cleanses will greatly enhance your we.
loss. It's perfectly fine to do a cleanse in tandem with the Fiber35 Diet; you can start
Phase One on the same day you start a fifteen- or thirty-day cleanse. In all the cases
look for a formulation that is delivered in vegetable capsules and contains no fillers
or binders (these are listed in the other ingredients section) like silicon dioxide or
microcrystalline cellulose. Always follow label instructions.

It's also important to take plenty of supplemental fiber when you are cleansing.
Soluble fiber supplements can be beneficial in removing toxins that have been
pulled from the organs and cells with herbs. Try to get an extra 5 to 10 grams of
soluble fiber in your diet every day during any herbal cleanse program.

Colon Hydrotherapy

As a colon therapist, I have practiced colonics for over fifteen years. A colonic is
basically an extended and more complete form of enema. Colon hydrotherapy
involves repeated infusions of filtered, warm water into all segments of the colon
by a certified colon therapist. Colon hydrotherapists are trained to use massage
techniques to help relax the abdominal muscles and ensure that all areas of
the colon are adequately irrigated and cleansed. Therapeutic benefits of colon
hydrotherapy include improved tone of colonic muscles, reduced stagnation of
intestinal contents, and reduced toxic waste absorption. While colon hydrotherapy
is not actually a weight loss procedure, it does often result in significant weight loss,
because of its ability to efficiently reduce the toxic burden of the large intestine.
Always look for a colon therapist who has been certified by the International
Association of Colon Hydrotherapy (I-ACT), and make sure that the therapist uses
FDA-certified equipment with disposable nozzles and filtered water.

As our world becomes ever more polluted, our bodies find it harder and harder to
cope with the accompanying toxins that are let loose into the environment. The
human body evolved in a natural setting and was designed to cope with common
environmental challenges. But with the help of cleansing herbs and a supportive
diet, we can be better prepared to deal with the unique challenges, particularly the
toxins, of modern life.

The Fiber35 Diet Detoxification Factor

- **There are basically two types of toxins:**

    External—those that enter the body from an outside source.

    Internal—those that are produced within the body.

- **Toxins can affect your ability to achieve your weight loss goals by:**

    Slowing your metabolism.

    Decreasing your ability to burn fat.

    Slowing down the satiety response.

- **To reduce the effects of toxins on weight loss, minimize toxins in your environment:**

    Eat organic foods when possible.

    Use natural household cleaners and body products.

    Install water and air filters.

- **Remove toxins from your body through:**

    Exercise

    Saunas

    Herbal cleansing

    Colon hydrotherapy

SUPPLEMENTS TO SUPPORT VIBRANT HEALTH

Throughout this book I've given guidelines regarding content and usage of a number of supplements that can help enhance your weight loss program. In this chapter, I'm going to offer a quick overview of this information, which is grouped into categories so that you may refer to it and access it readily.

It's not necessary to take every supplement described below. Many supplements are optional, depending on your individual condition, situation, and preferences. The information offered in each category and on each supplement is designed to help you tailor your supplement program to your personal needs.

Reminder: As with all the programs in this book, I recommend consulting your physician and sharing your plans with him or her before starting any supplement program. You may, for example, be taking prescription medication that can potentially conflict with ingredients contained in some of these supplements. I also suggest that you read product labels carefully and use products as directed. Because there are many manufacturers of supplements today, two formulas created for the same effect may have a different combination of ingredients, so it's impossible to provide specifics on dosage, or on how much of a given supplement to take and when. What I offer here is a general overview of formulas and ingredients—basic knowledge that you can then take to your physician and local health food store. I encourage you to find a trusted supplier of supplements; and if you're visiting a brick-and-mortar store, please don't be afraid to ask questions and seek the advice and recommendations of those who are familiar with a particular brand or product. If you experience any unusual side effects or want further help in tailoring the right supplement regimen to your body, start with your physician and consider seeking the advice of a local naturopathic professional as well. If you go to www.fiber35diet.com, you'll find further guidance in obtaining high-quality supplements as well as updated information on resources.

HEALTH MAINTENANCE SUPPLEMENTS

This category of supplements is designed for everyone, regardless of weight.

Omega-3 Fatty Acids

Taking a good-quality fish oil supplement will provide you with the omega-3 fatty acids you need to burn stored fat and eliminate excess omega-6 fatty acids, especially those from processed foods that are overconsumed in the standard American diet.

Of the many brands of fish oil on the market today, how do you choose the best? First and foremost, you'll want to look for a high-quality fish oil product that supplies a concentrated amount of the two important omega-3 fatty acids: EPA and DHA. I recommend selecting high-potency fish oil capsules that deliver 300 milligrams (mg) of EPA and 200 mg of DHA. One capsule per day of this potency is sufficient for most needs, though you may take three or more capsules to maximize your omega-3 intake. You'll want your fish oil capsules to be enteric-coated and formulated with the enzyme lipase. The enteric coating ensures that the contents of the capsule will not be released until it reaches the intestines. This may have other benefits as well; a study published in the *New England Journal of Medicine* concluded that enteric-coated fish oil supplements were effective in reducing the rate of relapse in Crohn's disease, a serious inflammatory bowel disease.[1] The addition of lipase to fish oil capsules aids in the digestion of the oil, as lipase is the enzyme needed for proper digestion of fats. If you tend to burp oils, a supplement containing lipase with an enteric coating can greatly reduce this effect.

Also, make sure that the fish oil you select has been tested for purity and is certified to be free of contaminants such as PCBs and mercury.

Multivitamin/Mineral

The key word here is *mineral.* You don't want just vitamins in your multi; you want a high-quality, well-formulated blend of vitamins and minerals. In selecting such a multi, look for a formula that contains a blend of mixed carotenoids as a source of vitamin A and important antioxidants.

Blood Sugar Support and Sugar Cravings

Unstable blood sugar levels constitute a formidable obstacle to weight loss. If you crave sugar, your blood sugar level may be unstable. If so, you will want to select a nutritional supplement formulated to naturally support insulin and sugar balance, one that features the minerals chromium GTF and vanadium, the amino acid L-taurine, and the herbs fenugreek seed, cinnamon bark, gymnema leaf, bitter melon, and jambolin seed.

Digestive Enzymes

Keeping your digestive tract healthy is important for proper digestion. Since your body's processing of food is central to metabolism and that utilization of energy, you can see how having an efficient digestive tract that can easily break down a variety of food can be key to weight loss efforts and an overall sense of well-being. There are numerous formulas that can help support your digestive tract, each one targeting a specific need. For example, if you're lactose intolerant and cannot digest milk products well, you may choose to seek a lactase supplement—preferably one that also contains lipase (to break down the fat) and papain (to break down the protein) that is also found in dairy products.

You don't have to be lactose intolerant, however, or deficient in a specific enzyme to benefit from a digestive supplement. You can also find formulas that offer a blend of several enzymes that, together, support your digestive functions in general no matter what kinds of foods you're eating (proteins, fats, carbs, and so on). And to help maintain a healthy intestinal lining, look for formulas that contain hydrochloric acid, pepsin, L-glutamine, N-acetyl-glucosamine, butyric acid, and probiotics. These are ingredients that your body needs to break down food and absorb essential nutrients.

FIBER SUPPLEMENTS

Ideally you'll be getting your 35 grams of daily fiber (or most of it) from fresh fruits, vegetables, legumes, whole grains, bars, and shakes. There will be times, however, when you'll want a quick, simple option for increasing your daily fiber intake. Your busy lifestyle may prevent you from eating three balanced meals every day, but there are ways to compensate when you have to grab a quick lunch while on the go or even when you miss a meal. Depending on your situation and personal preference, you may want to select one or more of the following fiber supplements.

Chewable Fiber Wafer

Eating a couple of chewable fiber wafers before one or more of your meals can help take the edge off your hunger, so that you eat less and still get your recommended daily allotment of fiber. These tasty wafers not only help satisfy your hunger but also displace higher-calorie food items. They can be easily stored and transported, so they offer a convenient option for supplementing your fiber intake when you are away from home. Ask you local health food store for help in finding these.

Chew fiber supplements before a meal. Add fiber in slowly to reach 35 grams. Should you become constipated, take a colon cleanse supplement before bed. It's really important to increase the water intake as you slowly add in the fiber. Also note that I do not recommend psyllium, because I have seen too many clients with too many complaints, like gas, bloating, and constipation.

Clear Fiber Supplement

Consider adding another shaker to your dinner table. Besides the salt and pepper shakers, you might want to keep a shaker full of soluble fiber on hand, preferably acacia fiber. This clear, tasteless soluble fiber can be sprinkled on your food liberally to enhance the fiber content of your meals without altering the taste. Best of all, it contains no calories!

Bulk Fiber Supplement

While not as convenient as the fiber supplements mentioned above, a powdered blend of fruit and vegetable fiber is a nutritious choice, for it is rich in important phytonutrients. A serving of such a product offers more fiber than acacia alone, and has the added advantage of containing both soluble and insoluble fiber, rather than just the soluble variety. Look for a powdered fruit and vegetable fiber supplement that has a fifty-fifty balance of soluble and insoluble fiber from a variety of fruits and vegetables, as well as other rich fiber sources like acacia gum, flaxseed, rice bran, guar gum, and larch fiber. Take this fiber blend as directed, adding a scoop to one 8-ounce glass of water. Taken before meals, this nutritious fiber blend can help decrease your appetite with minimal calories and prevent you from overeating in addition to supplementing your fiber intake. Or if you reach the end of your day and you are short on the recommended 35 grams, you can take a scoop before bed.

BARS AND SHAKES

Fiber bars and shakes are an integral part of the Fiber35 Diet, for you'll be taking two of each daily in Phase One and one each daily in Phase Two, as meal substitutes. Again, your local health food stores should be able to provide you with help in finding these types of bars and shake mixes.

Bars

The high-fiber bars you'll want to use will ideally contain 10 grams of fiber from milled flaxseeds, oat fiber, and acacia; and 10 grams of protein from whey protein concentrate. Whey is an extremely high-quality protein, complete with all essential amino acids. Look for a bar that is sweetened with dates, raisins, and agave syrup and comes in a variety of flavors. Avoid any bars containing hydrogenated vegetable oils. Look instead for high-oleic sunflower oil, a stable oil that is rich in essential fatty acids.

Shakes

You want your shake to provide 10 grams of fiber (from acacia) per serving. Because it is largely substituting for a meal, it should contain plenty of protein (20 grams) from a rich source, such as whey, as well as an array of important vitamins and minerals and an enzyme blend designed to ensure digestion of all classes of foods. Avoid any shakes that contain artificial sugar substitutes. Look for those containing tasty and nutritious natural sweeteners such as xylitol and stevia extract instead.

Chapter 10 Summary

Supplements to Support Vibrant Health

The supplement regimen recommended in this chapter is summed up in the chart below.

Required Supplements	Optional Supplements
Omega-3 fatty acids (fish oil)	Colon cleansing
Multivitamin and mineral	Improved rest and sleep
Calcium and magnesium (for women only)	Adrenal and energy support
Thermogenic weight loss formula	Blood sugar support (sugar craving)
Formula to increase lean muscle mass	Detox kits: 15-day, 30-day
	Supplemental fiber
	chewable wafers
	clear fiber (in shaker)
	fiber bars
	fiber shakes
	powdered fruit and vegetable fiber

CHAPTER 11

FIBER AND DISEASE PREVENTION

For many of my clients, changing their diet isn't just a matter of weight loss. It's also a matter of feeling better, having more energy, and getting relief from digestive problems like constipation and acid reflux. For Shirley, who was seventy-one, something struck her when she heard me say, "It's never too late to start taking care of yourself." She took those words of inspiration to heart and decided to do something about the state of her health from that day forward.

At five feet two inches and 164 pounds, Shirley was overweight, was often constipated, and suffered from acid reflux. No sooner did she start to change her diet and supplement properly on my program than she resolved her digestive ailments as the weight came off. And, like other clients, she enthusiastically reported how great she felt: "I did not feel like I was being punished as many diet plans make you feel. I dislike the word 'diet' and did not feel like this was restrictive in any way. I've lost 30 pounds so far and feel wonderful. The fiber amount in the Fiber35 plan also resolved my constipation problem, helping me to lose even more weight. I've finally learned a way to eat that's healthy and satisfying and keeps the weight off. If I gain a pound or two on a vacation to Italy, as I do at least twice a year, then I just go back through the plan's first two phases and lose the weight fast and simply."

Results like Shirley's really get me excited. I love hearing about people's medical transformations. While the weight loss aspect of the Fiber35 Diet is important, to me the most valuable aspect of this diet is the protection it can provide against disease, as well as the relief it can provide for current problems. I believe that those who ultimately succeed in reaching and maintaining their optimum weight have made a choice to live a new life that focuses on improving one's health, not managing one's weight. When you think about it, being overweight is really a symptom of not placing the highest value on one's health. Who among us has not taken health for granted? Our good health is something we earn, especially as we get older. Making a commitment to maximizing your quality of life as you age is the greatest gift you can give to yourself, an act of self-love and love for your family. There is nothing wrong with being motivated to lose weight so that you look great, but being motivated to maximize your health and life span gives you the will to maintain your weight for a lifetime. The Fiber35 Diet is an optimum health tool for two reasons:

1. **As a single ingredient, fiber is an incredible fighter against chronic diseases.**

2. **Fiber is found in foods that are tremendous disease fighters.**

Together, these reasons are very powerful for great health and disease prevention, and it is very important to understand the formula. The truth is that you have the power to take control of your health and use the wonders Mother Nature provided to ensure and protect your most valuable asset—your health.

Researchers agree that fiber reduces the risk of:

- **Digestive diseases**

- **Cardiovascular disease**

- **Heart attack**

- **High cholesterol**

- **Peripheral arterial disease**

- **Diabetes**

- **Cancer**

In this chapter, we're going to explore such issues as they relate to dietary fiber.

FIBER AND DIGESTIVE DISEASES

Digestive diseases are becoming increasingly common, with as many as 80 million Americans suffering from one kind or another. Fortunately, fiber helps prevent and correct many of them.

Constipation

This isn't a topic anyone likes to bring up at the dinner table, but constipation is one of the most common digestive complaints. More than 4 million Americans suffer from frequent constipation, accounting for more than 2.5 million physician visits each year. Unfortunately, constipation is a source of embarrassment that causes many who suffer from it to remain silent about their condition, and never seek help from a physician or an alternative practitioner.

The medical community cannot seem to agree on how many bowel movements per week are "regular," or how few constitute constipation. Alternative practitioners believe that you should have one to three good bowel movements per day. There are many causes of constipation, including diet, hormonal balance, and side effects of medication. Fortunately, fiber can help prevent constipation in the first place, and can return someone who is constipated to regularity. Fiber adds bulk to waste in the intestines, promoting the wavelike contractions that keep waste moving through the intestines.

In 1995, researchers at the Division of Digestive Diseases, Johns Hopkins Bayview Medical Center in Baltimore, performed a study to analyze the effect of fiber supplementation on physiology, mechanisms, stool parameters, and colonic transit times in a group of constipated patients.[1] Patients were given either a 24-gram fiber supplement or a placebo. Fiber supplementation appeared to benefit the constipated patients, reducing the time it took for waste to move through the colon from 53.9 hours to 30 hours. That's a difference of nearly 24 hours—a whole day.

Diverticulosis

This disease of the colon develops when the wall weakens and a pouch forms, protruding outward. Each pouch is called a diverticulum. Approximately 10 percent of Americans over age forty and 50 percent of those over age sixty have diverticulosis. There are many uncomfortable symptoms, including:

- **Bleeding (of the colon)**
- **Bloating**
- **Abdominal pain**
- **Cramping**
- **Diarrhea**
- **Constipation**
- **Gas**

Although not conclusively proven, the dominant theory is that too little dietary fiber and an associated condition, constipation, cause diverticulosis. Essentially, the pockets form when, over time, too much pressure in the colon weakens the colon wall, which then eventually expands outward. This disease is common in developed nations where fiber intake is low, but is rare in regions like Africa and Asia where fiber intake is high.

According to studies at Harvard University, those who eat more fiber are less likely to experience diverticulosis.[2] And for those who have the condition, fiber may help ease uncomfortable symptoms. The reason is that fiber lowers the pressure inside the large intestine, or colon, allowing bowel contents to move through more easily.

Gallbladder Disease

The gallbladder is a pear-shaped organ that sits under the liver. Its primary function is to secrete bile, a fluid that helps in digestion. Gallbladder disease is a swelling of the gallbladder, and this occurs most commonly when gallstones develop. A gallstone is a concentration of the components of bile, the primary component being cholesterol. Eighty percent of gallstones are of the cholesterol type, and are called cholesterol stones. The other 20 percent are called pigment stones, and they are made primarily of bilirubin and calcium salts. The most common symptom of gallstones is extreme pain, usually in the upper abdominal area, but someone with gallstones can also experience pain in the back. Anyone who has ever had gallstones would implore you to take every measure you can to avoid them.

Perhaps the best way to prevent gallstones is a high-fiber diet. Researchers at Harvard University also found a link between high-fiber diets and the reduction of gallbladder disease, particularly with a high intake of soluble fiber.[3] This makes sense, in that fiber can reduce the level of cholesterol in the blood, and the majority of gallstones are cholesterol-based.

Gastroesophageal Reflux Disease: GERD

Gastroesophageal reflux disease (GERD) is more commonly known as acid reflux disease, or heartburn. This condition occurs when liquids from the stomach are regurgitated into the esophagus. This liquid, in addition to causing significant discomfort, can, over time, damage the lining of the esophagus. In the past, researchers have attributed heartburn to a diet with large portions and a lot of fat, and to eating soon before bedtime. Now researchers are looking at the relationship between heartburn and fiber intake. In a study conducted at the Houston Veterans Affairs Medical Center, 371 people with GERD were questioned about the onset,

"AS NEEDED" SUPPLEMENTS

Not everyone is likely to need all the supplements listed below. Pick and choose the ones suited to you if you need support in any of these areas.

Colon-Cleansing

If you suffer from constipation, you'll want to select a well-formulated, nonirritating natural product to support colon function, one that will gently stimulate peristalsis, as well as hydrate, cleanse, and lubricate the intestine. Even if constipation wasn't an issue for you before you began the Fiber35 Diet, your bowel function may become sluggish once you start increasing your fiber intake, particularly if you do so too rapidly or fail to drink enough water. In this case, remember the guidelines for selecting an all-natural, effective colon-cleansing product. Choose one that contains ingredients like magnesium hydroxide, okra, triphala, and aloe.

Improved Rest and Sleep

If you have difficulty falling asleep at night or trouble staying asleep, the lack of rest can impair your weight loss efforts, as well as negatively affect your overall health and interfere with your ability to function optimally throughout the day. You can effectively regulate your sleep cycles without resorting to drugs that can produce many negative side effects. When you are choosing an all-natural rest product, remember to look for one containing calming minerals like calcium and magnesium, as well as antistress B vitamins (niacin and inositol), mild sedative herbs (like valerian root, passionflower, hops, chamomile, lemon balm, and skullcap) and 5-HTP, the precursor to serotonin, the neurotransmitter that helps you sleep.

Adrenal and Energy Support

If you are often under a lot of stress or you are lacking in energy, on both, your adrenal glands are going to need extra nutrional support. Without it, cortisol production goes unchecked and can result in unwanted weight gain. As discussed elsewhere in this book, ingredients for adrenal support include the B vitamin pantothenic acid (B_5), the amino acid L-theanine, and the herbs banaba, *Rhodiola rosea*, ashwaganda, and eleuthero root.

You'll want a formulation that includes the full spectrum of B vitamins, including the activated forms of B_2 and B_6 (riboflavin 5'-phosphate and pyridoxal 5'-phosphate, respectively).

You'll also want a multi that includes vitamin D_3, vitamin C, and vitamin E. Make sure that the vitamin E is in the form of d-alpha tocopherol. Avoid the "dl" form, which is synthetic. You'll want a high-potency vitamin C (about 1,000 mg) provided by ascorbic acid. An additional form of vitamin C, ascorbyl palmitate, a fat-soluble antioxidant, can enhance the formula.

Where minerals are concerned, in addition to the macrominerals (those needed in large amounts), such as calcium and magnesium, you'll also want to select a formula that has a wide range of trace minerals (those needed in small quantities), such as selenium, vanadium, chromium, boron, and iodine. Take these with meals according to label directions.

Calcium/Magnesium

Women have an extra need for these minerals, so they would do well to add a calcium-magnesium supplement containing the proper ratio of these important macronutrients. Look for a calcium-magnesium chelate containing a 2:1 ratio. This would be taken in addition to your multivitamin/mineral formula. Men need not add this additional supplement.

Supplements to Enhance Weight Loss

A central theme throughout this book has been how to rev up your metabolism to boost weight loss and how to decrease fat, while increasing lean muscle. To aid you in these efforts, you're going to want to look for two separate formulations, which I described in Chapter 7:

- **A thermogenic supplement containing such ingredients as iodine, tyrosine, banaba, and green tea extract.**

- **One that contains CLA (conjugated linoleic acid), banaba extract, and medium-chain triglycerides that will increase the ratio of lean muscle mass to fat.**

frequency, and severity of their symptoms, and about their diet over a yearlong period. The researchers discovered an inverse relationship between fiber intake and GERD. In other words, those who ate more fiber suffered less from GERD, and those who ate less fiber suffered more.[4] The lesson: if you suffer from heartburn, try eating more fiber!

Hemorrhoids

Perhaps there is no more embarrassing subject than hemorrhoids. However, this condition is extremely common in both men and women; about 50 percent of the population have hemorrhoids by age fifty. A hemorrhoid is a condition in which the veins around the anus or lower rectum become swollen and inflamed. Although physicians do not agree on the exact causes of hemorrhoids, most do agree that persistent straining in order to have a bowel movement can cause them. A high-fiber diet creates a soft bulky stool that passes easily. This type of stool helps prevent constipation and the need to strain to eliminate. More bulk means less pressure in the colon, and this may help avoid hemorrhoids.

FIBER AND CARDIOVASCULAR DISEASE

Over 50 million Americans suffer from cardiovascular problems. In fact, cardiovascular disease is the number one cause of death in the United States—for men and women. Cardiovascular disease is really a catchall phrase for a number of diseases that involve the heart, arteries, and veins. Usually cardiovascular disease refers to atherosclerosis, a disease of the arteries.

For example, in coronary heart disease, the arteries that supply blood to the heart become narrower, primarily because of a buildup of plaque made up of fatty deposits. Eventually, blood flow is severely restricted—much as a clogged sink in your bathroom slows the flow of water. This uncomfortable condition is called angina, and in the acute stage of this disease the plaque breaks off and forms a clot. That's when the blood flow to part of the heart is partially or completely cut off. As a result, that part of the heart begins to die. We call this situation a heart attack or, in more technical terms, a myocardial infarction.

Cardiovascular disease isn't confined to the heart; it can also affect the brain or the extremities. If you get a blood clot in any of your brain's arteries that stops the flow of blood, you suffer a stroke. Similarly, blood clots can form in the arteries that supply the arms or legs; this condition is called peripheral artery disease.

There are many risk factors for cardiovascular disease. The leading factors include:

- Age
- Poor diet
- Obesity
- High blood pressure
- Smoking
- Diabetes

Even though men are at higher risk than women, cardiovascular disease is still the number one killer of women, and women's risk after menopause is nearly equal to men's. It's no coincidence that we are experiencing an epidemic of cardiovascular disease at the same time that we are consuming far too little fiber. Large studies have shown that when you eat plenty of fiber, your risk of cardiovascular problems drops significantly.

When researchers at Harvard analyzed the results of several studies that collectively looked at the dietary habits of more than 330,000 people, they found that for every 10 grams of fiber consumed daily, the risk of a heart attack drops by about 14 percent.[5] Those 10 grams of fiber also reduce the overall risk of dying from some form of cardiovascular disease, including stroke, by 27 percent.

Another study, conducted at Tulane University in New Orleans, found that you can significantly lower your risk of heart disease by increasing your fiber by a mere 5 grams a day, the amount in one medium apple, ½ cup of peas, 2 tablespoons of flaxseeds, or a banana. In this research, which tracked the dietary habits of 10,000 people for twenty years, those who ate 20 grams of fiber a day, which is 5 grams more than the daily average for Americans, suffered fewer heart attacks.[6]

When researchers look at how consuming fibrous fruits and vegetables affects cardiovascular health, the results are equally impressive. In a nationwide dietary survey, the National Health and Nutrition Examination Survey (NHANES I), started in the 1970s, researchers began to study the diets of more than 9,600 people between ages twenty-five and seventy-four. Then, in the following decades, they charted the subjects' health and changes in diet and lifestyle. When the researchers examined how food choices affected the risk of cardiovascular disease and stroke, they found that eating high-fiber foods was remarkably protective. Eating fruits and vegetables at every meal lowered the risk of heart problems and kept people alive significantly longer.[7]

The statistics in this study indicated that three servings a day of fruits and vegetables may reduce the risk stroke by 27 percent (that's a 9 percent reduction with every apple). Those three servings also may reduce the risk of dying from a stroke by 42 percent (more than 13 percent per serving). The risk of heart disease may drop by 27 percent, and the risk of dying from heart disease may shrink by 24 percent. Although this study found in general that men benefited more than women from a high-fiber diet, both sexes derived strong health advantages. In fact, a woman's chance of death from a stroke dropped by 53 percent when she ate a fiber-rich diet of fruits and vegetables.

Researchers believe that, as impressive as those numbers are, they may actually understate the benefits of a high-fiber diet rich in fruits and vegetables. Why? Because this study measured only up to three servings a day, as opposed to the recommended five or more. Eating even more fibrous foods probably produces an even greater benefit.

FIBER HELPS KEEP ARTERIES CLEAR

In the summer of 2005 the *American Heart Journal* reported evidence that a "high-fiber diet may slow atherosclerosis," which is the buildup of plaque in the arteries.[8] American and Finnish researchers were looking at the effects of whole grain fiber on 229 postmenopausal women who already had blocked arteries. The "modestly smaller declines in coronary artery blockage" found in women consuming larger quantities of fiber indicate that fiber not only may help prevent heart disease but may also be beneficial to those already affected by heart disease.

Cholesterol Reduction   *(OATMEAL)*

One way fiber helps fight heart disease is by improving the type of cholesterol that circulates in your blood. Cholesterol has gotten a lot of attention in recent years, and for good reason. Too many people are walking around with high cholesterol, especially high levels of the "bad" LDL type that's more strongly linked to heart disease. Drug companies have been working overtime to formulate and market drugs that can lower cholesterol, and today's statins are among the hottest-selling drugs. But they are still drugs, and a natural way to control cholesterol is almost always the better alternative.

Cholesterol is a pliable, waxy material that the body uses to make cellular membranes and protect structures such as nerves. Cholesterol travels around the blood in chemicals called lipoproteins. High-density lipoproteins (HDL) are called good cholesterol; they transport cholesterol to the liver, where it is broken down.

Low-density lipoproteins (LDL), so-called bad cholesterol, are associated with the deposit of cholesterol on artery walls. Once there, these deposits form plaque that, as I just mentioned, can block blood flow and result in heart attacks and strokes. If a blood test shows your LDL to be over 160 milligrams per deciliter (mg/dL), you are considered to be at an increased risk of heart disease.

In research presented at a conference of the American Heart Association, scientists reported that fiber supplements lower LDL while raising protective HDL. In this 3-month study, HDL rose by more than 20 percent while LDL dropped by almost 30 percent. Fiber was also found to help decrease triglycerides (blood fats), which are linked to cardiovascular complications. These fell by 14 percent.[9]

Some experts have gone as far as to argue that fiber can act as miraculously as cholesterol-lowering drugs. William R. Davis, MD, author of *Track Your Plaque*, states, "In addition to LDL lowering effects, fiber smoothes out spikes in blood sugar that carbohydrates cause. This reduces triglycerides and even blocks the development of diabetes." He goes on to suggest that "increasing your daily fiber intake to 35 grams or greater (is) nearly as good as the cholesterol lowering drugs."[10]

Because fiber lowers cholesterol, it may help prevent heart attacks. This effect is the result of soluble fiber binding with bile acids, which digest fat and contain toxins, and removing them from the body.

Fiber, Cholesterol, and Heart Health

When cholesterol builds up in the artery walls, your risk of blood clots, heart attacks, and stroke is greatly increased. But the truth is that having too little cholesterol in the blood can also lead to health problems. Here again, the key is balance. We need saturated fat found in animal products, but eating too much of it can adversely affect our heart health. To keep your intake of saturated fat down to a moderate level, avoid fatty meats and choose lean beef, chicken, or fish as your major source of protein.

A steady daily helping of fiber also is crucial. For every 10 grams of fiber you consume every day, your risk of a heart attack may drop by about 14 percent.[11] Those 10 grams of fiber may also reduce the overall risk of dying from some form of cardiovascular disease, including stroke, by 27 percent.

Blood Pressure

Another risk factor that contributes to heart problems is high blood pressure, also known as hypertension. Today, hypertension runs rampant in North America, and like obesity, is increasing worldwide. About one in three Americans currently suffers from hypertension. Globally, about one in five people have it. By the year 2025, about 1.5 billion people are expected to be hypertensive.[12]

While obesity has been identified as an imminent serious global epidemic, cardiovascular disease as a result of hypertension has also been on many medical experts' radar. "The global burden of high blood pressure supports predictions of a worldwide epidemic of cardiovascular disease," notes Jiang He, MD, PhD, a professor of public health at Tulane University who has studied the spread of hypertension. "During the past century, such disease has changed from a minor cause of death and disability to one of the major contributors to the global burden of disease. Cardiovascular diseases are now responsible for 30 percent of all deaths worldwide."

But the good news is consuming more fiber can help. Research at Tufts University in Boston found that feeding people more fiber, in this case from oats, reduced their systolic blood pressure by an average of 7 points in six weeks.[13] (Blood pressure is expressed as a ratio of systolic pressure to diastolic pressure. Systolic is pressure exerted as the heart beats. Diastolic is the residual pressure between beats. A healthy blood pressure is less than 120/80.) When food is digested more slowly, levels of insulin rise more slowly. Insulin, a hormone released by the pancreas during digestion, helps regulate the absorption of sugar, but when it's secreted too quickly it can also send blood pressure skyrocketing. Fiber tempers this process.

A FIBER35 DIET SUCCESS STORY

Sandee is a lot like millions of others. She tried many diets in the past and had struggled to lose those last 10 to 20 pounds since high school. She found herself in a constant yo-yo pattern: dropping the weight, then gaining it back plus more. And she was a sugar junkie, thinking about ice cream and cake all the time. When she turned fifty, her doctor informed her at an annual physical that her blood pressure was in a pre-hypertension state and that medications should be considered. Sandee didn't want medications. She didn't want to go down a path that would lead to other drugs, which she'd then have to rely on for life. Instead, she wanted to take charge of her health once and for all, and find a way to eat that would work for her in the long-term. So she went on the Fiber35 Diet and discovered a friend for life. The craving for sugar stopped, and Sandee began to lose an average of 2 pounds a week while eating small meals every three to four hours. Sandee is close to her goal weight (if not already there by the time you read this) and looks forward to reintroducing reasonable portions of ice cream and cake into her diet occasionally during the last phase. No drugs needed!

Smoking

Don't expect me to endorse smoking; you know it's one of the worst things you can do to your health. And I won't give you a lecture on the health risks associated with smoking. But I do want to share some astonishing research that shows how high-fiber diets may help blunt the effects of smoking and other risk factors for heart disease. If you're a victim of secondhand smoke, listen up!

A Finnish study, published in 1996, involved 21,903 male smokers age fifty to sixty-nine, who were divided into two groups: one eating a high-fiber diet, and the other eating a low-fiber diet. The men whose fiber intake was high (averaging 35 grams daily) had one-third fewer heart attacks than those whose fiber intake was low (15 grams daily). The risk of dying from heart disease decreased by 17 percent for each 10 grams of fiber consumed by these men.[14]

In the United States, a study involving 43,757 male health professionals (some of whom were described as sedentary or overweight, or were smokers, or both) found that those consuming more than 25 grams of fiber per day had a 36 percent lower risk of developing heart disease than those who consumed less than 15 grams daily. The risk of dying from heart disease was also lowered—by 29 percent for each 10 grams of fiber consumed.[15]

Adults who eat more than 7.5 grams of fiber a day—the equivalent of two apples a day—are less likely to have health effects associated with childhood exposure to secondhand smoke.[16]

FIBER AND THE FIGHT AGAINST DIABETES

Type 2 diabetes, also called adult-onset diabetes, is striking Americans in record numbers. Surely you've heard the outcries from public health institutes hoping to put a stop to the spread of this epidemic. According to the National Center for Chronic Disease Prevention and Health Promotion, it is the sixth leading cause of death in the United States and afflicts more than 18 million people. As the U.S. population (on average) ages and gains weight, the incidence of this debilitating disease continues to climb. But here's a bit of positive news: simply increasing the fiber in your diet can lower your risk of this pernicious, largely preventable disease.

Type 2 diabetes, the most frequent type of diabetes, occurs when the body loses its ability to keep blood sugar levels under control. Insulin is supposed to encourage cells to take sugar out of the blood. When diabetes is present, the body becomes insulin-resistant, unable to respond to insulin's efforts to reduce blood sugar.

The complications of diabetes can threaten one's life and can lead to amputations, blindness, and an increased risk of Alzheimer's disease and kidney damage. Nerve damage linked to diabetes is particularly insidious, since there is no treatment for it. Known as peripheral neuropathy, this damage can cause numbness, deep pain, and weak muscles. Research shows that it can occur when bone marrow cells malfunction. These cells begin to produce insulin. They then migrate out of bone tissue, latch onto nerve cells, and kill them. The result is irreversible, and painful.[17]

Daily Habits

Many of our daily habits promote diabetes. Lack of exercise and being overweight significantly raise your risk. So do smoking and a diet that lacks fiber. Let me share with you some real data that illustrate how our lifestyle choices affect our risk of diabetes.

Our Daily Bread

When researchers looked at the eating habits of more than 40,000 male health professionals over age forty, they found that those who ate whole grains like brown rice, dark breads, and whole grain cereals had a significantly reduced risk of diabetes. In this study, men who ate the most fibrous foods (three or more servings a day) reduced their risk of diabetes by over 40 percent! Those who were obese, but still exercised, developed diabetes 50 percent less than obese people who were inactive.[18]

Another study, involving 65,000 women over a period of six years, demonstrated that indulging in processed foods, sugary soft drinks, and other fiberless items such as doughnuts, white rice, and white bread more than doubles the risk of diabetes. On the other hand, merely eating whole grain cereal for breakfast reduces the risk of diabetes by 28 percent! Those are impressive numbers. Is fiber really the miracle ingredient that separates the doughnuts from the dark breads—the diets that can lead to obesity and diabetes from the diets that can optimize your health? I wholeheartedly believe so.

I explained earlier that one reason for the benefits of fiber is its ability to slow the movement of food out of the stomach. That gradual release of food in the presence of fiber slows the absorption of glucose into the blood, enabling a controlled insulin response. As glucose trickles slowly into your bloodstream, your pancreas gets a break because it doesn't have to pump out enormous quantities of insulin to tame a flood of foods high in sugar and low in fiber. So your overall level of blood sugar remains steady. In addition, the magnesium found in whole grains also tempers the body's response to glucose and insulin. The result? The body's blood sugar balance is better and the insulin-making machinery of the pancreas experiences less stress.[19] Translation: you reduce your risk of diabetes.

It's been widely reported that obesity and diabetes often go hand in hand; obesity is the single most important risk factor for becoming diabetic.[20] The combination of diabetes and obesity has been dubbed diabesity, and lo and behold, it's been a subject of studies that show how fiber helps us take off weight and controls blood sugar.

In one study, four obese men with diabetes were placed on high- and low-fiber diets of 800 calories a day.[21] While on these diets, the men reported before and after each meal on their hunger and feelings of fullness. Not surprisingly, the high-fiber diet proved more filling and more satisfying. In another experiment, twenty-five people were switched to a high-fiber diet, and they all experienced more control over blood sugar as they lost weight. In fact, their blood sugar balances were better during the two-and-a half-years of follow-up. On average, they managed to maintain 56 percent of their weight loss.[22]

These types of studies clearly demonstrate that fiber can increase weight loss, reduce hunger, and result in better overall health. (But by this point I may have already convinced you of that!) It's no longer a theory that fiber may support blood sugar balance and in turn reduce one's risk for diabetes. It's now a fact confirmed over and over again by scientists.[23] High-fiber diets, coupled with cutting calories, take off pounds. With exercise, you can lose even more weight. I should also add that a healthy blood sugar balance also means less body fat is created. Steady insulin levels translates to a more efficient body, much like a car running on a steady flow of premium gasoline.

If you are one of the millions of Americans who have type 2 diabetes, you should strongly consider adopting a high-fiber diet and exercising, once you have consulted your physician. A high-fiber diet can decrease the frequency and quantity of blood sugar swings, help to lower blood pressure, and improve your overall cholesterol. All these benefits may in turn decrease your risk of diabetes-related disorders such as blindness, nerve damage, and heart disease. You may even be able to reverse the severity of your diabetes; studies are now showing dramatic medical transformations among diabetic—and even prediabetic—people who lose considerable weight, normalize their blood sugar balance naturally, and no longer need medications to treat their conditions.[24] Talk about medical transformations! More proof that you hold the key to unlocking a lifetime of vibrant health.

Although the benefits of fruits and vegetables for the bones may be linked to their potassium and magnesium, researchers cannot rule out other factors, such as fiber, as an aid to bone strength. An important discovery in the study was that people who ate large amounts of processed foods lacking in fiber and minerals had weaker bones. Eating a diet low in fiber also makes you more likely to be among the almost 30 million Americans who suffer from osteoporosis, a degenerative bone disease that often occurs in middle age, resulting in broken hips which in many cases cause disability and a generally downward health spiral.

THE STRENGTH OF FIBER

Are you convinced yet? Just as the phrase *moral fiber* refers to a person of upstanding character who can withstand temptation, the fiber in food helps our bodies stand up to disease. Although I encourage you to adopt the Fiber35 Diet in order to look your best, I wrote this book to help you feel your best now and in the future. As well as being your secret formula for controlling weight, a high-fiber diet provides you with incredible advantages that help you to prevent and fight against some of the most common and most serious health concerns of our time. If you know people who do not need to lose weight but are not eating a high-fiber diet, I encourage you to share your newly acquired knowledge with them. They, too, deserve the benefits found in this miraculous diet!

Chapter 10 Summary

Fiber and Disease Prevention

- **Fiber and Digestive Diseases**

    As many as 80 million Americans suffer from digestive diseases.

    Fiber is extremely useful in the management of constipation, diverticulosis, gallbladder disease, gastroesophageal reflux, and hemorrhoids.

- **Heart Health and Cardiovascular Disease**

    For every 10-gram increase in fiber, the risk of heart attack drops by 14 percent.

    A high-fiber diet may slow atherosclerosis.

    Three servings per day of fruits and vegetables may reduce your risk of stroke by 27 percent and your risk of heart disease by 27 percent.

    Fiber can lower your LDL cholesterol, raise your HDL cholesterol, and lower your triglycerides.

    A high-fiber diet helps to reduce blood pressure.

    Thirty-five grams of fiber per day can lower the risk of heart attack in smokers.

- **Fiber and Diabetes**

    Increasing fiber intake can lower the risk of type 2 diabetes and help stabilize blood sugar.

- **Fiber and Cancer**

    High-fiber diets protect against colon cancer.

    Diets rich in at least five servings of cruciferous vegetables per day may lower the risk of pancreatic cancer.

    Diets rich in fruits, vegetables, fiber, and olive oil may lower the risk of gastrointestinal cancer.

    High-fiber diets protect against breast cancer.

- **Fiber and Other Disease**

    High-fiber diets may protect against Alzheimer's disease.

    Diets rich in fruit and vegetables support strong bones.

THE POWER OF PHYTONUTRIENTS

During the past ten years, scientists have made astounding discoveries about vegetarian foods. Such foods contain a remarkable number of natural chemicals that help the human body fight disease and achieve optimal health. These substances can apparently fight the effects of aging, decrease muscle soreness, lower your risk of arthritis, help defend against heart disease and cancer, and protect the brain against the damage that leads to Alzheimer's disease.

For much of the twentieth century, food scientists focused most of their attention on vitamins—the micronutrients found in food that are necessary for survival. When your diet is missing a particular vitamin, over time you will suffer from a vitamin deficiency disease that can threaten your life. For example, in the past when we traveled by boat, limes were brought along for a vital supply of vitamin C, the lack of which can cause scurvy and eventual death.

Knowledge of the necessity and power of vitamins has been widely established for decades, but more recently, researchers have discovered thousands of other phytonutrients that have an incredibly powerful effect on our health. It is as if we have discovered that there are really thousands of vitamins, not just the handful we all know about. These phytonutrients are found primarily in fruits and vegetables, as well as tea, nuts, whole grains, and legumes. Some phytonutrients owe their power to their antioxidant ability to destroy free radicals. Free radicals, which are known to destroy cellular structures, are thought to be involved in causing or complicating diseases like cancer and heart disease. Harmful free radicals can result from exposure to pollution and other toxins, as well as being produced by the body as it goes about its daily metabolic processes.

In Chapter 3, I briefly outlined the power of phytonutrients—plant chemicals that aid in a plant's own survival. Put simply, plants use phytonutrients to protect themselves from disease and to boost their own immunity. When we eat plants we gain some of the same benefits in those phytonutrients. That's one reason researchers believe organic fruits and vegetables are healthier—they are raised without pesticides, and this forces them to produce more of their own protective chemicals. When we eat organic produce, we reap the benefit of the natural chemicals that plants have originally made for their own protection.

Let me give you an example. The phytonutrients in apples include chemicals called phenolic acids that defend the fruit against viruses, bacteria, and fungus. In this group of phenolics, a large family of chemicals that include the flavonoids, is a natural antioxidant called quercetin that protects apples against disease. Research at Cornell University shows that consuming quercetin (which is mostly contained in apple skin and just below the peel) may lower the risk of Alzheimer's disease and Parkinson's disease by defending nerve cells against damage by free radicals.[1] In addition, previous studies have shown that quercetin helps the body fight off cancer. Is this proof that an apple a day keeps the doctor away? I think we're just beginning to understand the power of these phytochemicals, and there will be nothing but good news ahead.

A whole book could be written on phytonutrients, but here I want to share with you a basic overview of the topic so you'll become familiar with their names and come to appreciate the foods you'll be choosing to nourish your body from the inside out.

TERPENES, PHENOLICS, THIOLES

The phytonutrients in apples are just the beginning of the phytonutrient story. The major groups of phytonutrients are called:

- **Terpenes, which include the chemicals that give food their colors: beta carotene makes carrots orange, lycopene makes tomatoes red, and zeaxanthin makes spinach green.**

- **Phenolics, which include the anticancer lignans in flaxseeds, the heart-protecting resveratrol in grape skins, and the anticancer isoflavones in soy.**

- **Thioles, which includes the sufide compounds in onions and garlic that help protect the cardiovascular system, and the tumor-fighting isothiocyantes found in cabbage, cauliflower, and broccoli.**

The Color Wheel

A simple guide to eating using phytonutrient colors was devised at the University of California to promote the consumption of a wide range of phytonutrients. If you eat at least one food from each of the following groups every day, you will ensure that you are getting a wide range of phytonutrients.

- **Green-yellow: avocado, spinach, mustard greens, green beans, and collard greens contain lutein and zeaxanthin, pigments that promote eye and heart health.**

- **Orange: squash, mangoes, apricots, carrots, pumpkins, and cantaloupe contain alpha and beta carotenoids, which help lower the risk of cancer.**

- **Orange-yellow: oranges, tangerines, pineapples, and other citrus fruits contain bioflavonoids, which promote cardiovascular health and lower the risk of cancer.**

- **Red-purple: grapes, red wine, strawberries, raisins, and cherries contain health-supporting compounds called anthocyanins, ellagic acid, and flavonoids, which support heart health and fight arthritis and muscle soreness.**

- **White-green: garlic and onions contain allyl sulfides, which promote healthy arteries.**

- **Red: tomatoes and watermelon contain lycopene, phytoene, and phytofluene, which help lower the risk of cancer.**

- **Green: broccoli, cauliflower, brussels sprouts, cabbage, and bok choy contain glucosinolates, isocyothianates, and indole-3 carbinol, which help fight cancer.**

Lycopene

Lycopene, the red pigment that gives tomatoes their distinctive color, has won great respect as a powerful antioxidant that defends against carcinogens. For instance, studies by German and Dutch researchers have demonstrated that lycopene inhibits the growth of prostate tumors. In these laboratory tests, combining lycopene with vitamin E created a potent anticancer weapon. Lycopene slowed the reproduction of prostate cancer cells by half; and when vitamin E was added, the combination reduced tumor growth by more than 70 percent.[2]

CANCER PROTECTION

Meanwhile, scientists at the Fred Hutchinson Cancer Research Center have conducted research demonstrating that lycopene is merely one anticancer phytonutrient in a world of anticancer phytonutrients. In their epidemiological studies, they have found that eating three servings of vegetables a day can cut a man's risk of prostate cancer by almost 50 percent. This study discovered that the most powerful anticancer phytonutrients were in cruciferous vegetables—cabbage, cauliflower, and brussels sprouts.[3] Those are convincing numbers.

What's so powerful about cruciferous vegetables? They contain sulforaphane (SFN), a chemical that's been shown to inhibit the effect of carcinogens. Researchers at Rutgers further found that vegetables rich in SFN might be able to forestall cancers that are genetically linked. Interestingly, they discovered that these compounds from broccoli, cauliflower, and brussels sprouts acted like gunfire against cancerous cells. When they exposed cancer cells to these phytonutrients, the cells self-destructed (technically, such self-destruction is called apoptosis). And adding turmeric, a spice that contains the phytonutrient curcumin, can enhance the anticancer effects.[4]

Garlic Power

Garlic, whose characteristic odor and flavor have made it a popular addition to the culinary repertoire, is a phytonutrient star among foods. The phytonutrients in garlic can help fight infection, improve cardiovascular health, and lower the risk of cancer. For example, if you like to barbecue in the summer, you can improve the safety of your steaks and other meat dishes by cooking them with garlic.

When high-protein foods like meat are cooked on a barbecue, they release a chemical known as PhIP, a toxic substance linked to cancer. (Studies demonstrate that women who eat large amounts of barbecued meat have a significantly increased risk of breast cancer.) However, a phytonutrient called diallyl sulfide (DAS), one of the sulfide compounds that give garlic its characteristic smell, can inhibit the carcinogenic effects of PhIP. DAS protects DNA from damage and stops the conversion of PhIP in the body into other carcinogenic substances. When researchers at Florida A&M University in Tallahassee treated breast cells of rats with PhIP and then added DAS, the garlic compound stopped the cancer process in its tracks.[5]

HEART PROTECTION

Can a steady diet of phytonutrient-rich meals lower your risk of heart disease more effectively than drugs? With tongue only partially in cheek, researchers at McGill University in Canada came up with the "polymeal," a combination of phytonutrient foods that could theoretically lower the risk of heart disease by more than 70 percent. According to these scientists, research demonstrates that eating meals every day that include fruits, vegetables, a glass of red wine, fish (four times a week), and dark chocolate could increase a man's life expectancy by 6.6 years. A woman eating the same foods could boost her life expectancy by about 5 years.[6] Adding tea to these meals could also heighten the benefits.

Although the scientists making this recommendation were not totally serious (medical professionals have reservations about recommending alcoholic beverages and chocolate), other researchers noted that the recommendation was actually based on sound research. For instance, dark chocolate has compounds that support cardiovascular health. And having a cup of flavonoid-rich tea with your chocolate enhances the heart-protective effect even more.

Flavonoids have gained a lot of fame recently as new science shows the benefits of getting a wide mix of these heart-friendly compounds for overall health. They are typically found in grapes, including grape juice and even red wine, and have been shown to reduce the oxidative stress that gives rise to cardiovascular problems. Furthermore, they can help protect cholesterol from being oxidized (a process that can block arteries) while guarding other cells and substances in the bloodstream from being damaged.[7]

PHYTOESTROGENS AND CANCER

In a growing body of research, scientists are also looking at how the phytonutrients called phytoestrogens can improve health. Phytoestrogens are natural substances that mimic the effect of estrogen, the female hormone. Although some cancers may be exacerbated by the body's own production of estrogen, researchers believe that phytoestrogens in food may reduce the risk of these same cancers. For instance, when researchers at the Anderson Cancer Center in Houston looked at data on the lung health of more than 3,400 people, they found that those who ate the most foods containing phytoestrogens had the lowest incidence of lung cancer.[8]

The phytoestrogens that produced the greatest protective effect included:

- **Isoflavones, found in soy foods, chickpeas, and red clover**

- **Lignans, found in carrots, spinach, broccoli, and flax**

- **Coumesterol, contained in spinach, beans, sprouts, and peas**

One puzzle in this study was the fact that men obtained more cancer protection from phytoestrogens than women did. But both sexes still benefited.

LET FOOD BE YOUR MEDICINE

As research continues on the thousands of health-promoting phytonutrients, even more benefits are bound to be discovered. That's why when the Institute of Food Technologists summed up its research on phytonutrients, its report recalled that more than 2,500 years ago, Hippocrates, the father of medicine, said, "Let food be your medicine and medicine be your food." Researchers admit that food as medicine is a topic which has only begun to be understood and appreciated.

Phytonutrient Anticancer Meal Plan

The Fred Hutchinson Cancer Research Center in Seattle, Washington, offers a sample menu to show how you can get plenty of phytonutrients in your daily meals and lower your risk of cancer. Notice the volume of fiber-rich produce in every meal and snack:

- **Breakfast: Drink a glass of tomato or other vegetable juice; eat a slice of tomato on toast; add sautéed vegetables to scrambled eggs or omelets.**

- **Lunch: Eat a salad with plenty of carrots, red cabbage, or other raw vegetables; include vegetable soups like beef vegetable, minestrone, or cream of broccoli soup; include a side dish of cooked vegetables.**

- **Dinner: Serve two vegetables with the main course or a vegetable and a salad; add vegetables like peas and spinach to (whole grain) pasta; combine several vegetables with casseroles.**

- **Snacks: Munch on raw vegetables like carrots, cherry tomatoes, celery, broccoli, or cauliflower florets and eat plenty of fruit.**

Chapter 12 Summary

The Power of Phytonutrients

- **Fiber-rich foods are loaded with natural chemicals called phytonutrients that protect us from disease.**

- **The phytonutrients that lend color to purple, red, orange, yellow, white, and green vegetables promote:**

    Increased immunity and lowered infection

    Eye and heart health

    Lowered risk of cancer

    Reduced arthritis pain and less muscle soreness

    Healthy arteries

    Liver detoxification

- **Phytonutrients:**

    In garlic, can protect from carcinogens in charbroiled meat

    Called phytoestrogens, can protect both men and women from cancer

    In apple skin, can protect against cancer and neurodegenerative disorders

    In chocolate and tea, can promote cardiovascular and artery health

- **Phytonutrients produce a broad range of beneficial health effects. In their most important actions they:**

    Stimulate cancer cells to self-destruct (in a process called apoptosis)

    Provide a source of vitamin A

    Enable cells to communicate more effectively

    Beneficially shift estrogen metabolism to lower the risk of estrogen-related cancers

    Boost immunity

    Offer antioxidant protection against free radicals

    Protect DNA against damage linked to pollution and tobacco smoke

    Activate enzyme systems that protect against carcinogens

HORMONES, STRESS, AND WEIGHT GAIN

Our understanding of the elusive interrelationship between hormonal balance and weight management has become clearer in the past two decades. It's difficult to talk about weight without addressing the topic of hormones. After all, if hormones had nothing to do with being fat or thin, then we probably wouldn't experience so many fluctuations in our weight, especially at pivotal points in our lives such as when we are growing teenagers; when we go through acutely stressful times; or when women, for example, go through menopause. A lot of research is currently under way, and more will continue to be conducted in the future, that will shed more light on this fascinating field of medicine.

We've already seen how appetite hormones correlate strongly with whether or not we're going to pick up that Danish. We've also covered the effect insulin has on blood sugar balance, which in turn affects how much fat the body creates. But there's much more to this topic that deserves our attention. In fact, the subject of hormones as they relate to the body and weight could be a book in itself, much like the subject of phytonutrients. For our purposes, we're going to briefly explore the six most powerful hormones that affect weight management so you can use what we currently know to reach your weight loss goals. Mere awareness of how these hormones directly or indirectly relate to weight control can help you make better decisions in your life to support your body's natural balance.

SIX HORMONES THAT CAN AFFECT WEIGHT MANAGEMENT
Chief among the many hormones that may affect your weight are the
following six: cortisol, insulin, thyroid T3 and T4, leptin, and estrogen.

CORTISOL AND STRESS

Stress is so commonly discussed today that many people may not be aware of the
large role it plays in weight management. What's more, stress can lead to many life-
threatening diseases while also playing a part in other maladies from the common
cold to arthritis and degenerative diseases. Basically there are three hormonal
stress responses: acute, chronic, and adrenal burnout. Acute stress that becomes
chronic can eventually lead to adrenal burnout—a condition you don't want.

From Harmless Acute Stress to Dangerous Adrenal Burnout

If you've ever had to take a serious test or speak in front of a very large group
of people for the first time, then you've certainly experienced acute stress. Acute
stress is also what people often feel before a physical test, such as running a
10-kilometer race, or at the moment they realize they're about to be in a car accident.
Other than the rush of anxiety and nervousness that fill you, you're probably
not aware of what's going on at the cellular level in your body. Well, a lot is
happening in a rapid sequence of events—starting from the very moment you
sense danger or the sudden demand for physical or mental performance. I'll give
you a short description.

First, the brain's hypothalamic center releases corticotrophin-releasing
hormone (CRH). This hormone then travels to another nearby area of the brain,
the pituitary, where it causes the release of adrenocorticotrophic hormone (ACTH),
which in turn travels through the body's circulation to the adrenals—the small
glands that sit on top of the kidneys. The adrenals then release three hormones.
The first two are epinephrine and norepinephrine, which increase heart rate and
cardiac output of blood, and selectively increase blood flow to the muscles, lungs,
and brain to allow for enhanced performance during the stressful moment. As
a result, your concentration becomes more focused, reaction time is faster, and
strength and agility increase. This is why you can feel a sudden rush of invincibility
when you're acutely stressed. The release of epinephrine and norepinephrine is
soon followed by a third hormone, cortisol, which helps raise blood sugar and calm
the body down in order to let it recover from the stressful event.

The point is that your body undergoes a chain of chemical reactions that help you get through the stressful event. But imagine having this reaction take place over and over again in the body. At some point it becomes chronic. And too much stress over long periods of time can eventually hurt you. Your body doesn't want to be in "fight or flight" mode all the time.

Ideally, the hormonal signals switch off the stress response and the body returns to normal when the stressful event is over. The problem comes when we cannot forget about the event, we continue to worry, and we allow other, smaller bothersome events to enter our mind. Chronic low-grade stress is rampant in our society today. Even the very technology that's supposed to make our lives easier and less stressful, such as the use of e-mail and cell phones, has somehow made us more stressed out as we lead 24/7 lives.

Unfortunately, in this chronic state, stress hormones continue to wash through the system at fairly high levels, never leaving the blood and tissues. The chronic elevation of cortisol can eventually cause the hypothalamic receptors in the brain to become insensitive and not transmit the clear message that there is plenty of cortisol in the bloodstream. The hypothalamus, rather than stopping the production of CRH, continues to release increased amounts of CRH that continue to elevate cortisol (in medical language this is known as loss of feedback inhibition).

This persistent elevation of both cortisol and CRH has negative effects on the body. For one, the increased cortisol can lead to insulin resistance, which promotes further fat deposition. It can also lead to diabetes, heart disease, stroke, and depression. What's more, the increased CRH can lead to the release of inflammatory messenger molecules (technically, TNFalpha, IL6, and IL1) that then lead to inflammation throughout the body. And, as you've learned, chronic inflammation can ultimately result in further fat deposition and depression.

The downward spiral doesn't end there. As chronic stress continues, the adrenal glands can eventually become fatigued and stop producing cortisol in response to CRH and ACTH. Cortisol levels that become too low cause adrenal burnout or exhaustion. This is serious because normal amounts of cortisol are needed to help control body pain, inflammation, blood sugar, blood pressure, fatigue, mood, and emotional stability. So no matter which end of the spectrum you're on—producing too much cortisol or too little—it's a lose-lose situation. You must achieve a balance of cortisol levels in your body to reap its rewards and avoid its pitfalls when it goes unchecked. And controlling your stress levels is exactly how you can arrive at this healthy balance.

I believe that stress is the most underemphasized and undermanaged threat to our health and our weight. Stress has become ubiquitous in today's society—a commonly accepted condition of living. When you're sitting in traffic, or watching horrors on the nightly news, or tending to your quarreling children, your body is potentially shifting into a survival mode that works against your best efforts to be lean and healthy. I often wonder how much healthier we'd all be if we lived in a stress-free world. I bet the statistics related to illnesses and disease would be vastly different.

THE FIBER35 DIET STRESS FORMULA

Because combating stress is so vital to your overall health, I've designed a Fiber35 Stress Formula. It has five components:

1. **Nutritional supplementation**

2. **Antistress diet**

3. **Exercise and sleep**

4. **Caffeine reduction**

5. **Meditation**

Nutritional Supplementation

Several nutritional ingredients and herbs help regulate cortisol production and support the adrenal glands. The relationship between vitamin B_5 (pantothenic acid) and the adrenal glands has long been evident. The adrenal glands depend on vitamin B_5. A deficiency of this vitamin puts continual stress on the adrenals, and such stress can eventually lead to exhaustion and malfunction of the glands. Herbs such as ashwagandha root, eleuthero root (ginseng), and *Rholiola rosea* are all considered adaptogenic; that is, these herbs have a history of supporting adrenal function and cortisol production as well as enhancing our ability to withstand the negative effects of stress. Products that use a potent, standardized extract of ashwagandha are more effective in controlling stress-related weight gain. Banaba extract, along with regulating blood sugar, has been shown to reduce cortisol production and support adrenal function. The amino acid L-theanine is believed to induce relaxation and relieve emotional stress, because of its ability to cross the blood-brain barrier and contribute to the production of GABA, an amino acid in the brain that acts like a chemical and is well-known for its calming effects. Look for these ingredients in a supplement designed to support adrenal and cortisol health.

Antistress Diet

By now you should know the best way to eat for weight loss and optimum health. So it shouldn't come as a surprise to you when I say that eating a daily diet high in organic plant foods (fruits, vegetables, legumes, nuts) reduces the physiological stress related to eating. What do I mean by *physiological stress related to eating*? Eating puts some stress on your body—mainly because the body has to do work to digest food. Here are some specific examples.

- **Processed and preserved foods: Consuming foods that are processed and loaded with preservatives may trigger immune reactions that create overall physiological stress.**

- **Improper combining of food: Too much protein (especially red meat) eaten at the same time as simple processed carbohydrates (bread, pasta, etc.) causes a reaction between the protein and carbohydrate to produce advanced glycation end products (AGEs). These are absorbed and cause a release of free radicals from the immune system that in turn produces further stress and inflammation. You can think of AGEs as something that "ages" you more quickly.**

- **Lack of enzymes: Cooked food is low in enzymes and therefore may not be digested properly, especially as we age. I encourage taking digestive enzymes, which I detailed in Chapter 10, to naturally support proper digestion.**

Exercise and Sleep Relative to Stress

It has been said that timing is everything, and so it is with stress, particularly stress related to exercise, sleep, and hormone production. A healthy diurnal (day-night) cycle is tied to our normal patterns of hormonal secretion. Cortisol should be highest in the morning and then progressively decrease throughout the day, with the lowest levels occurring after 11 p.m. With low evening cortisol levels, melatonin levels rise. Melatonin is your body's natural hormone that tells you it's time to sleep. Higher melatonin levels will allow for more rapid eye movement (REM) sleep, which helps maintain healthy levels of growth hormone, thyroid hormone, and male and female sex hormones. In fact, growth hormone is released mostly at night, when you're filling your sleep bank with high-quality, restful sleep. This is the hormone necessary for cellular repair and rejuvenation. If you miss out on deep sleep, not only will you feel sluggish and not refreshed the next day, but your body will have missed out on getting its much-needed levels of growth hormone.

Since most exercise tends to increase cortisol, it would make sense to exercise earlier in the day. This allows for cortisol to decrease before bedtime, and that decrease supports your normal sleep cycle. (That said, let me reiterate that you should worry less about finding the ideal time of day to exercise and more about finding any time at all. Late-day exercise is best for some, and they have no problem getting to sleep at night. Go with what suits your individual needs.) Inadequate sleep and low hormone production occur when the cortisol pattern is flipped (high cortisol at night and low in the morning). The flipped cortisol pattern has been shown to be a strong predictor of death in cancer and heart patients.

Moderate exercise has profound anti-inflammatory and antistress effects, whereas heavy, prolonged exercise releases huge quantities of stress hormones and keeps cortisol levels high for hours. For this reason, I recommend moderate levels of exercise. Does this mean that you shouldn't do an hour of cardio? No. It means that you shouldn't be pushing yourself to exhaustion every time you work out. Listen to your body. It will tell you when the time has come to stop.

As we have already discussed in Chapter 7, getting proper sleep is one way to boost your metabolism. Sleep is equally important with regard to to your hormonal balance.

GOOD NIGHT TIP: AVOID LATE-NIGHT TELEVISION AND YOUR COMPUTER SCREEN

Getting a full night's sleep is hard for many individuals, but it's vital to your overall health. Watch out for late-night light exposure when your body wants to go to sleep, especially exposure from a television or computer screen. The light emitted can send faulty light signals to the brain from the retina of your eyes, both increasing cortisol and decreasing melatonin. You then become alert and won't want to sleep. And your hormones won't be in proper balance. If you must be in front of a television or computer screen, you can try wearing rose-colored glasses, which have been shown to blunt the effect. But on a more practical level, just get to bed!

Caffeine Reduction

Caffeine can be another culprit that raises our cortisol levels. Does this mean that you need to avoid coffee altogether? That's up to you. But a better alternative to coffee would be caffeinated tea. And if you are going to drink coffee, it's best to do so early in the day. Everyone metabolizes caffeine at a different a rate, but in general it takes approximately three to seven hours for the body to eliminate half of the total amount of caffeine (also called the half-life). The longer caffeine remains in your bloodstream, the longer cortisol may be raised. In one study, measuring the effect of 300 mg of caffeine taken before 1 p.m., cortisol levels returned to normal by 7 p.m.[1]

Meditation

We all know that physical exercise is good for the body, but what about exercise for the mind? Meditation is a form of exercise for the mind, providing a way to relax and release built-up stress. The history of meditation goes back even farther than that of yoga. Meditation brings together all the energies of the mind and focuses them on a chosen point: a word, a sound, a symbol, an image that evokes comfort, or one's own breathing. Reports show that the blood chemicals indicative of a stressful state decrease during periods of meditation. I meditate every morning on waking or in the evening after a stressful day and find that it greatly helps my state of mind, allowing me to deal more easily with stressful situations. Getting the proper meditation chair is important. I prefer the Seagrass Meditation Chair because it provides great back support during my meditation sessions. (See the Resource Directory for information.)

STRESS MANAGEMENT TIP: CONSIDER COUNSELING AND READING ENLIGHTENING MATERIAL

Stress management can also come in the form of counseling and reading enlightening material. Beyond exercise, diet, restful sleep, and meditation, counseling and reading enlightening or spiritual books and articles can help reframe our interpretation of stressful events so that they will have less an impact on our emotions, thus mitigating the release of the stress hormones.

INSULIN

Low-carbohydrate diets are built primarily around insulin, which has been an important concept in weight loss in recent times. This is because we now have a better sense of how fluctuations in this commanding digestive hormone can affect weight and our overall health. Insulin is, after all, a definitive factor in diabetes. By now you should have a basic understanding of this hormone as it relates to blood sugar balance and weight management. Although I do not believe in low-carb diets, I do believe that controlling insulin is important, and it can be done with the right carbohydrates.

Insulin-Balanced Nutrition

The key to insulin-balanced nutrition is to avoid carbohydrates that cause a rapid rise in blood sugar and a surge of insulin—otherwise known as high-glycemic foods. As I noted in Chapter 5, the glycemic index measures the rate at which foods are converted into blood sugar. The higher the glycemic index rating of a food, the faster this conversion to sugar takes place, and the more insulin response is required to manage sugar levels in the blood. This index should not be relied on entirely in making food choices, but it can help you differentiate the good from the bad carbs, since refined and processed carbohydrates tend to be high on the index.

Avoid "bad" carbs that include refined carbohydrates such as:

- **Chips (corn, potato, etc.)**

- **White breads that are not whole grain**

- **Pasta that is not whole grain**

- **White rice**

- **Candy, cakes, and pastries**

- **Most fast foods**

- **Most fried foods**

- **Sugary sodas and drinks**

- **Sugary cereals**

In contrast, sticking to the good, low-glycemic carbs will help balance your insulin. Good carbs are essential to health and are naturally fiber-rich. They include:

- **Fruit**

- **Vegetables**

- **Legumes** (Beans)

- **Whole grain breads and pasta**

- **Brown rice**

NUTRITIONAL SUPPLEMENT TIP: LOOK FOR AN INSULIN–BLOOD SUGAR FORMULA

There are natural nutritional ingredients that help support insulin and sugar balance. Chromium—specifically chromium glucose tolerance factor (GTF)—has been recognized since the 1970s as an essential nutrient for glucose tolerance and insulin stability. The mineral vanadium is known as an antidiabetic agent because of its insulin-like effects in the body. Herbs such as fenugreek, cinnamon bark, gymnema leaf, bitter melon, and jambolin seed have been clinically shown to lower high blood sugar and help maintain healthy levels. The amino acid L-taurine is believed to have the effect of improving insulin resistance. One study found that insulin resistance was lower in a test group that used taurine as a supplement. Look for a combination of these ingredients when you are choosing an insulin support supplement.

THYROID T3 AND T4 HORMONES

Your weight is greatly affected by your thyroid, which regulates your metabolism, the rate at which you burn calories for energy. Reduced thyroid activity causes your metabolic rate to decrease. The result is that food is not properly assimilated and eliminated, and low thyroid quite often leads to unnecessary weight gain. Hypothyroidism results from the underproduction of the two thyroid hormones T4 (thyroxine) and T3 (triiodothyronine). Signs and symptoms may include any of the following:

- Weight gain
- Headaches
- Fatigue
- Loss of appetite
- Depression
- Low blood sugar
- Increased adrenaline and cortisol
- Elevated cholesterol
- Heart disease
- Blood pressure irregularities
- Poor circulation
- Intolerance of cold
- Decreased body temperature
- Chronic infections
- Insomnia
- Emotional distress
- Dry skin and hair
- Premature graying of hair in young adults
- Swollen eyelids
- Decreased heart rate
- Lack of libido
- Immune deficiencies
- Constipation and other colon problems

Don't be alarmed if you have many of the above symptoms; your physician can do a simple test to check your thyroid. The medical treatment for hypothyroidism most often includes thyroid hormone replacement with synthetic T4.

Before taking any supplements that may affect your thyroid, check with your physician to determine if you have hyperthyroidism. Some supplements may exacerbate a hyperthyroidism condition.

The best nutritional ingredients traditionally used to support thyroid health include iodine, tyrosine, banaba, and DMAE. If you choose to take a natural thyroid support formula, these are the ingredients to look for. Many of these ingredients are found in thermogenic and insulin-support nutritional supplements.

LEPTIN

Our understanding of appetite-regulating hormones like leptin and ghrelin has vastly improved in just the last few years. In late 2004, for example, researchers showed the strong connection between sleep and the ability to lose weight; the more one sleeps, the better the body can regulate the chemicals that control hunger and appetite. One of these hormones is leptin, which, as you'll recall, is made by fat cells and is responsible for telling your brain that you are full. When functioning normally, it induces fat burning and reduces fat storage. Obviously, you want this hormone to be working properly so that its counterpart—ghrelin, the "feed me" hormone—will stay under control.

In 1994, ten years before the breakthrough studies on sleep and appetite hormones came out, *ob gene* was identified in genetically obese mice. It was found that mutations in the ob gene caused a total lack of leptin production, leading to severe obesity. Scientists further discovered that when leptin was injected into these mice, their food intake decreased, their metabolic rate increased, and they lost a significant amount of weight. This research seemed promising until a study found that obese humans had leptin levels that were on the average four times higher than individuals of normal weight, suggesting that human obesity does not correlate with a lack of leptin production and so cannot be successfully treated with leptin injections.[2] Nonetheless, research on the hormone continues, and recent clinical trials have found evidence that leptin can result in weight loss in obese individuals. Research has also shown that exercise may normalize your body's sensitivity to leptin.[3] So perhaps it's not a lack of leptin but rather a condition of leptin resistance—similar to insulin resistance—that influences obesity in humans. I predict that we will understand more intricacies related to obesity and these hormones with future research. We are just breaking the surface, and it's an exciting time in this area of research.

High-Fructose Corn Syrup Signals Sky-High Cravings

High-fructose corn syrup has largely replaced sugar as the sweetener of choice in today's processed foods. And it's more harmful to your weight loss goals than you probably think. Aside from the fact it's a highly processed sugar high in calories and with little nutritive value, it can actually mess with your ability to determine when you should stop eating. How? Leptin will not be secreted so much in the presence of high-fructose corn syrup. So it can't deliver the all-important message to your brain that you're full. And as a result, you can't stop eating.[4] The obvious lesson here is that any product made with high-fructose corn syrup should be strictly avoided by anyone trying to lose weight.

Soluble Fiber and Leptin

In August 2006 a study published by the University of California, San Francisco, determined that a diet high in calories and low in fiber promotes hormonal imbalances that encourage overeating.[5] In particular, too much sugar and too little fiber appear to be the main causes of the obesity epidemic, through their effects on insulin and leptin. Insulin and leptin share a central pathway, and it seems that insulin functions as a leptin antagonist. Too much sugar and not enough fiber will promote an overabundance of insulin, which in turn will block the signal of leptin to the brain, resulting in increased food intake and decreased activity. With this information at hand, one might assume that by regulating the production of insulin with a reduced-sugar and high-fiber diet, you may restore the brain's sensitivity to leptin.

Earlier in 2006, scientist found that leptin levels could be normalized by adding to the diet a soluble fiber, which could then improve insulin sensitivity.[6]

ESTROGEN

Virtually every woman will admit feeling the effects of estrogen (and probably also progesterone, estrogen's "sister hormone"). But not every woman knows how far-reaching estrogen's effects on the body can be—especially when estrogen levels become imbalanced. An elevated estrogen level can lead to a sluggish metabolism, paving the way for weight gain. Higher levels can also cause your body to hold onto sodium, resulting in water retention, as well as change the way your body metabolizes the amino acid tryptophan, a precursor to the feel-good neurotransmitter serotonin.[7] If your serotonin levels drop, you can experience powerful cravings for unhealthy foods (you'll seek comfort foods, which are usually high in fat, salt, and low-quality carbs in order to artificially produce that feel-good sensation). Those cravings will be likely to lead you down a path to weight gain.

Additionally, when estrogen dominates over progesterone, you can put yourself at greater risk of developing breast cancer, as well as hypothyroidism. Hypothyroidism develops when your metabolism-regulating thyroid downshifts into a less active state, thus inhibiting your weight loss efforts.[8]

While it's difficult to point out exactly what causes imbalances in estrogen and progesterone, especially since every woman's body is different and is exposed to a different environment, all women should aim to achieve a balance that may help prevent certain kinds of cancer and promote ideal weight management. A starting point for supporting that healthy balance simply can include adding more fiber to the diet.

Fiber and estrogen may seem to be a world apart, but there is a proven relationship between high fiber intake and decreased estrogen levels in the blood. I mentioned that fiber is believed to reduce excessive estrogen by binding to it in the colon, which ultimately eliminates it from the body in the stool. Conversely, in a low-fiber diet estrogen is reabsorbed and recycled in the body, increasing the body's overall levels of estrogen, which can then potentially feed tumor growth. Excess estrogen may reach the breasts and other organs vulnerable to hormone-related cancer. So by taking a healthy dose of fiber, you can potentially get rid of an unhealthy dose of estrogen.

There's a lot more to estrogen hormonal balance than fiber alone, but my point in bringing this up is to suggest that shifting from a low-fiber, high-processed diet to a high-fiber, nutrient-rich diet can afford you many health benefits—benefits beyond those provided by the fiber itself—and thus can ultimately bring your body into a more balanced, healthy state.

Chapter 13 Summary

Hormones, Stress, and Weight Gain

- **There are several hormones that affect weight management:**

    Cortisol

    Insulin

    Leptin

    Thyroid

    Estrogen

- **The Fiber35 Diet Stress Formula will help you to support hormonal balance and optimum weight management through:**

    Nutritional supplementation

    Antistress diet

    Exercise and sleep

    Caffeine reduction

    Meditation

CHAPTER 14

THE FIBER35 RECIPES

The following recipes offer a variety of some of my favorite meals, many of which take minimal time to prepare. Many of these recipes are full meals and include ingredients such as fresh fruits and vegetables to provide a higher fiber content per serving. Some recipes are simply ideas on how to cook chicken or fish. These are to be used as your protein source; then add a vegetable recipe or two to complete the meal. I have also included recipes for salads, soups, and the shake drink suggested in Phase One and Phase Two of the plan, as well as snacks that contain both fiber and protein. All these recipes can be included in Phase One, Phase Two, or Phase Three of the Fiber35 Diet Plan. You'll find these recipes organized into sample menus in Chapter 15.

All these recipes have been designed to work with any phase of the diet. Every individual's daily caloric requirements will be different, so you have to focus only on creating meal plans that match your personal needs. None of these recipes contains more than 500 calories per serving (and most contain much less). For example, during Phase One you can select any recipe here, but just make sure you still remain within your calorie budget for each day. If you choose the 483-calorie vegetable lasagna for dinner, for instance, you must work this around your other calories for the day and go for lower-calorie options for breakfast and lunch. It's doable and it's easy! Simply plan ahead, and you will succeed.

Look carefully at the serving sizes of the recipes, as these will vary. You can always adjust the ingredients down for serving one or two, or up for a family-size gathering.[1] I have included some tips and notes that may be helpful when you are preparing the meals.

Remember that you can increase the amount of fiber per serving of any of these recipes by sprinkling table fiber directly on your meal before eating. This type of fiber is clear, tasteless, and odorless and should not alter the taste of the recipe in any way. Visit www.fiber35diet.com for more diet tips and ideas.

BREAKFAST RECIPES

MULTIGRAIN FRENCH TOAST WITH YOGURT AND BANANAS

serves two (6g fiber/serving)

- 1 whole egg and 1 egg white, lightly beaten
- ¼ teaspoon real vanilla
- Pinch of salt
- Pump spray olive oil
- 4 slices of nutty organic whole grain bread
- ½ cup banana, sliced
- 2 medium figs, sliced
- 6 ounces of plain yogurt

Combine eggs, vanilla, and salt in a bowl large enough to lay 1 piece of bread in it flat. Preheat a skillet to medium and spray with oil. Set 2 pieces of bread in your egg mixture, coating both pieces well on all sides. Hold the bread in the egg mixture to soak up roughly half of the egg. Place the bread into the heated skillet and cook until slightly golden brown on both sides. Repeat for the remaining 2 pieces of bread. Plate the French toast then top with a big spoonful of yogurt, banana and fig slices.

Note: Whole grain breads vary in nutritional content. Make sure to use whole grain bread, not just a multigrain.

Brenda's Tips: The type of bread used in this recipe can make a big difference in the taste. Breads with grains, nuts, seeds, and even added vegetables and fruits can often be found at health food stores.

Nutrition Facts: Serving size, 2 slices—calories 295, fiber 6 g, protein 14 g, fat 7 g, saturated fat 3 g, carbohydrate 47 g, cholesterol 104 mg, sodium 400 mg, sugars 22 g.

MILLET PORRIDGE

serves two (7g fiber/serving)

- ½ cup dry millet*
- ¼ cup almond milk
- ½ teaspoon cinnamon
- ⅛ cup almonds, chopped**
- ¼ cup fresh raspberries
- 1 teaspoon maple sugar (looks like brown sugar)
- 1 teaspoon SweetLife or other natural sugar substitute (if needed)
- Dash salt

Soak millet overnight covered in water in a large bowl. In the morning, drain soaking water and rinse.

Bring 1½ cups of fresh water (lightly salted) to boil. Add millet, stirring frequently. Reduce heat to simmer and continue to cook for approximately 15 minutes or until all liquid has been absorbed by the millet. Remove from heat. While the millet is still very warm, add ¼ cup almond milk, cinnamon, and almonds and return to heat for about 2 minutes. Spoon into serving bowl. Sprinkle with raspberries and maple sugar. Add sugar substitute to sweeten to taste.

*Note: *If millet is presoaked, the cooking time is shortened by 5 to 10 minutes. The grain has a fluffier texture when less water is used and is very moist and dense when cooked with extra water.*

***All nuts should be soaked overnight.*

Brenda's Tips: I love this recipe as an alternative to oatmeal. Millet is a highly nutritious, non-glutinous food. It is considered one of the least allergenic and most digestible grains.

Nutrition Facts: Serving size, 1 cup—calories 262, fiber 7 g, protein 8 g, fat 6 g, saturated fat 1 g, carbohydrate 45 g, cholesterol 0 mg, sodium 29 mg, sugars 4 g.

SALMON FRITTATA

serves two (5g fiber/serving)

- 1 teaspoon (extra-virgin) olive oil
- ¼ cup (sweet) onion, diced
- ¼ cup frozen or fresh steamed corn kernels
- One 4-ounce can of salmon, drained
- 1 (vine) tomato, diced
- ¼ cup red bell pepper, chopped
- 1 whole egg and 1 egg white, lightly beaten
- 4 cups raw fresh spinach
- ¼ cup avocado, sliced
- ¼ cup of your favorite salsa
- 1 tablespoon fresh mint or basil, chopped
- Pinch of sea salt
- Freshly ground black pepper
- Optional: 3 tablespoons cheddar cheese

In a heavy skillet heat olive oil over medium heat. Cook onion until softened or light in color. Add corn, salmon, tomato, and bell pepper. Gently stir to combine and continue to cook for about 4 minutes. Pour eggs over the mixture. Cook at medium heat for about 4 minutes. Remove skillet from stovetop and place under a broiler until light golden brown. Cut frittata into wedges and serve on a bed of spinach topped with fanned avocado slices and salsa. Sprinkle with fresh herb, salt, and pepper. Sprinkle with cheddar cheese if desired.

Note: You may use Bibb lettuce or mixed greens instead of spinach. Most of the fat in this recipe is the good essential fats from avocado.

Brenda's Tips: This is my favorite quick and easy meal for breakfast, lunch, or dinner. I especially love it because it's easy when company drops in unexpectedly. Plus, it's so easy to make vegetarian.

Nutrition Facts: Serving size, 1 wedge—calories 260, fiber 5 g, protein 23 g, fat 13 g, saturated fat 2 g, carbohydrate 15 g, cholesterol 146 mg, sodium 347 mg, sugars 6 g.

SPINACH AND CHÈVRE (SOFT MILD GOAT CHEESE) OMELET

serves one (3g fiber/serving)

- ¼ cup chèvre (goat) cheese
- 2 teaspoons (extra-virgin) olive oil
- 2 cups firmly packed, fresh, whole-leaf spinach
- ¼ cup sweet onion, diced
- 4 ounces frozen artichokes, thawed and roughly chopped
- 1 whole egg and 3 egg whites, lightly beaten
- Salt and pepper to taste

Combine eggs in a mixing bowl. Reserve 1 teaspoon chèvre cheese for topping. Heat 1 teaspoon of olive oil in 9-inch skillet over medium-high heat. Add spinach to the skillet and, using tongs, flip often. Cook spinach for only a few minutes, until most leaves are slightly wilted, then remove spinach from skillet and place in a bowl.

Heat remaining 1 teaspoon of olive oil in same 9-inch skillet and reduce heat to medium. Add onion and artichokes and sauté for 2 minutes until vegetables are slightly tender.

Add eggs, and while cooking gently lift edges to let the wet egg slide under. Cook for approximately 3–4 minutes, until the egg is firm enough to flip. Flip omelet and immediately spread chèvre on top. Cover with warm wilted spinach and continue to cook for approximately 2 minutes on low heat.

Fold in half and remove from skillet. Cut omelet in half and plate. Dollop with reserved spoonful of chèvre. Season with salt and pepper to taste.

Note: If you do not like goat cheese, 2 ounces of another type of cheese can be substituted. To reduce the fat in this recipe, you can use an olive oil pump or spray in place of the 2 teaspoons of olive oil.

Brenda's Tips: This omelet is so quick and easy that you can make it during the busy workweek.

Nutrition Facts: Serving size, ½ omelet—calories 220, fiber 3 g, protein 17 g, fat 14 g, saturated fat 6 g, carbohydrate 9 g, cholesterol 119 mg, sodium 335 mg, sugars 2 g.

BLUEBERRY ALMOND AND FLAX BUCKWHEAT PANCAKES

serves two or three (7g fiber/serving)

- ½ cup almond flour
- 2 tablespoons ground flax meal
- 1 tablespoon baking powder
- 1 tablespoon buckwheat flour
- 1 teaspoon Sweetlife or other natural sugar substitute
- ¼ cup almond milk
- 1 egg yolk
- ¼ cup vegetable oil
- 2 egg whites
- Pump spray olive oil
- ½ cup (fresh) blueberries
- 1 tablespoon maple syrup

In mixing bowl, combine flour, flax, baking power, buckwheat flour, and sugar substitute. Slowly incorporate almond milk, egg yolk, and vegetable oil into dry ingredients. In a separate bowl beat egg whites to soft peaks. Fold beaten egg whites into pancake mixture. Heat a large skillet over medium heat and spray lightly with olive oil. Gently ladle the pancake batter into skillet to make approximately a 5- to 6-inch round. Sprinkle blueberries onto pancake rounds. When bubbles begin to set around the edges of the pancake and the griddle side of the cake is golden, gently flip the pancake. Continue to cook 2–3 minutes or until the pancake is set. Remove from skillet, plate, and serve with maple syrup. Repeat with remaining batter.

Note: Most of the fat in this product is good essential oils from flax, almond, and buckwheat. The flours suggested can be found at your local health food market. If you have difficulty finding either of the flours suggested, then whole wheat flour can be substituted.

Brenda's Tips: To reduce the sugars by half, try using a light whipping cream with vanilla extract instead of maple syrup for the topping.

Nutrition Facts: Serving size, 3 pancakes—calories 326, fiber 7 g, protein 13 g, fat 20 g, saturated fat 1 g, carbohydrate 28 g, cholesterol 105 mg, sodium 596 mg, sugars 13 g.

STEEL-CUT OAT CRUNCH

serves one (12g fiber/serving)

- ½ cup dry steel-cut oats
- 1 cup water
- ½ teaspoon sea salt*
- ½ Granny Smith apple with skin, chopped
- ¼ cup almond milk, plain
- ¼ cup chopped raw walnuts**
- Cinnamon to taste

Mix the oats, water, and salt in saucepan; cover; and let soak overnight.*** In the morning, heat the oat mixture over medium heat until creamy, approximately 5–10 minutes. Remove from heat; stir in chopped apple, almond milk, and walnuts. Pour into serving dish and sprinkle with cinnamon to taste.

Notes: * To reduce sodium, exclude the sea salt.
**All raw nuts should be soaked overnight.
*** Soaking the raw oats overnight will decrease cooking time by 20 minutes.

Brenda's Tips: This breakfast will stay with you throughout the morning. Steel-cut oats are a much better, healthier choice than rolled oats.

Nutrition Facts: Serving size, 1 cup—calories 312, fiber 12 g, protein 8 g, fat 14 g, saturated fat 1 g, carbohydrate 42 g, cholesterol 0 mg, sodium 620 mg, sugars 8 g.

FRESH FRUIT PARFAIT

serves one (10g fiber/serving)

- ¼ cup (fresh) strawberries, sliced
- ¼ cup (fresh) blueberries
- 1 Granny Smith apple with skin, cored and chopped
- ¼ cup raw almonds,* chopped
- 1 teaspoon ground cinnamon
- ½ cup plain yogurt
- 2 mint leaves

In a mixing bowl fold fruit, nuts, and cinnamon into yogurt. Serve in small glass dish. Garnish with mint leaves.

Note: All sugar is derived from fruit sources in recipe.

*All nuts should be soaked overnight.

Brenda's Tips: Try preparing enough fruit and nuts ahead of time and keeping them stored in the refrigerator for easy preparation in the morning. If cow's milk is a problem, substitute goat yogurt. If apple peel bothers you, peel the apple and add ground flaxseeds for fiber.

Nutrition Facts: Serving size, entire recipe—calories 351, fiber 10 g, protein 12 g, fat 19 g, saturated fat 3 g, carbohydrate 40 g, cholesterol 15 mg, sodium 55 mg, sugars 26 g.

SHAKE RECIPES

Shakes are a great way to satisfy hunger pangs and get a delicious, filling, nutritious blend. They are also quick and easy to prepare. Of course, I'm not talking about ice cream shakes or shakes that contain chocolate syrup. You'll find the shake blends that I'm referring to in your local natural health food store. Many large, traditional grocery chain stores are beginning to offer more organic products and brands typically found in health food stores, but you may have a hard time finding these nutritious shake mixes in your regular supermarket. If this is the first time you've ever tried to find these shake mixes, don't worry. You can take this information to your local health food store and someone will be able to guide you in the right direction. These powder mixes usually come in a canister with a small spoon inside to help you measure out the proper number of scoops. Follow the directions on the label. You'll find mainly chocolate and vanilla varieties, and you may want to experiment with different brands (and flavors) to find the one that you enjoy the most.

The calorie amount per shake may vary slightly, depending on the brand of shake mix you choose. For these recipes I am using one that contains approximately 160 calories along with 10 grams of fiber and 20 grams of protein per serving. That's what you should aim for when seeking a suitable shake mix.

You can make up your own recipes using any type of fruit, nut butter, or other ingredients. Be creative and delicious, but keep the calories under 250 to fit into your meal planning during Phase One and Phase Two.

RASPBERRY DELIGHT

serves one (14g fiber/serving)

- Vanilla shake mix
- ½ cup frozen raspberries
- 4 ounces almond milk
- 4 ounces water

Using an electric blender on medium setting, blend all ingredients together and serve in tall glass.

Nutrition Facts: One serving—calories 220, fiber 14 g, protein 21 g.

ORANGE PINEAPPLE CRAVE

serves one (10g fiber/serving)

- Vanilla shake mix
- ½ cup frozen pineapple chunks
- 4 ounces orange juice
- 4 ounces almond milk

Using an electric blender on medium setting, blend all ingredients together and serve in tall glass.

Nutrition Facts: One serving—calories 280, fiber 10 g, protein 20 g.

CHOCOLATE BANANA DREAM

serves one (12g fiber/serving)

- Chocolate shake mix
- ½ frozen banana
- 4 ounces almond milk
- 4 ounces water

Using an electric blender on medium setting, blend all ingredients together and serve in tall glass.

Nutrition Facts: One serving—calories 250, fiber 12 g, protein 20 g.

CHOCOLATE PEANUT BUTTER BANANA BLITZ

serves one (12g fiber/serving)

- Chocolate shake mix
- 1 teaspoon chunky peanut butter
- ½ frozen banana
- 8 ounces water

Using an electric blender on medium setting, blend all ingredients together and serve in tall glass.

Nutrition Facts: One serving—calories 285, fiber 12 g, protein 22 g.

CHOCOLATE MOCHA MADNESS

serves one (10g fiber/serving)

- Chocolate shake mix
- 8 ounces almond milk
- 1 teaspoon decaf instant coffee
- Dash of ground cinnamon

Using an electric blender on medium setting, blend all ingredients together and serve in tall glass.

Nutrition Facts: One serving—calories 225, fiber 10 g, protein 20 g.

SALAD RECIPES

BIG SALAD

serves two (10g fiber/serving)

- ½ tomato
- ¼ cup cucumber, sliced
- ¼ cup endive, cut into thin strips
- ¼ cup small white beans, canned, rinsed
- ¼ cup garbanzo beans, canned, rinsed
- 3 radishes, sliced thin
- ¼ cup red onion, chopped
- 3 cups mixed baby greens: arugula, romaine, radicchio, mesclun, spinach—red and green leaf
- ¼ cup carrots
- 2 ribs celery, chopped
- ¼ cup fennel, sliced
- ¼ cup raw almonds*
- 1 tablespoon raw sunflower seeds
- Optional: 3 tablespoons of your favorite low-calorie dressing

Toss first eleven ingredients. Top with nuts and seeds. Finish with your favorite dressing (optional).

*Note: *Soak almonds overnight.*

Brenda's Tips: I love making salads at the beginning of the week so that I can have them available as a side dish to any meal. This one makes a great lunch, and look at the fiber!

Nutrition Facts: Serving size, ½ recipe—calories 300, fiber 10 g, protein 13 g, fat 16 g, saturated fat 1 g, carbohydrate 30 g, cholesterol 0 mg, sodium 53 mg, sugars 5 g.

GREENS AND BEANS SALAD

serves two (12g fiber/serving)

- 1 tablespoon fresh minced cilantro
- ½ tablespoon chopped fresh parsley
- ½ tablespoon fresh lime juice
- Salt and pepper to taste
- ¹One-half 15-ounce can no salt black beans, rinsed and drained
- ½ cup chopped tomato
- 1 ear fresh corn (taken from cob)
- 1 tablespoon red onion
- ½ tablespoon chopped, seeded jalapeño pepper
- 2 cups salad greens

Combine first four ingredients in a bowl with a whisk. Add beans, tomato, corn, onion, and jalapeño pepper; toss well. Cover and chill 2 hours or—better—overnight.

Serve over salad greens.

Brenda's Tips: I love this salad as a side dish, or with tortilla chips as a salsa.

Nutrition Facts: Serving size, ½ recipe—calories 216, fiber 12 g, protein 12 g, fat 1 g, saturated fat 0 g, carbohydrate 43 g, cholesterol 0 mg, sodium 13 mg, sugars 2 g.

LAYERED BLACK BEAN SALAD

serves six (17g fiber/serving)

- 2 tablespoons olive oil
- 6 tablespoons fresh lemon juice or lime juice
- 3 tablespoons rice wine vinegar
- 1 tablespoon Dijon mustard
- Fresh ground pepper
- 12 cups baby spinach leaves, stems removed, loosely packed
- 3 cups cherry or grape tomatoes
- 1 medium yellow bell pepper, seeded, cut into quarters, and sliced thin
- 1 medium red bell pepper, seeded, cut into quarters, and sliced thin
- Two 15-ounce cans low-sodium or no-salt black beans (drained and rinsed)
- 4 ounces shredded reduced-fat sharp cheddar cheese
- 1 medium avocado, peeled, pitted, and sliced into ½-inch pieces

To make the dressing, in a small bowl whisk together olive oil, lemon or lime juice, vinegar, mustard, and pepper. Set aside.

In a deep, clear, glass bowl, layer the salad as follows: 6 cups spinach leaves, 1½ cups tomatoes, ½ yellow bell pepper, ½ red bell pepper, 1 cup beans, ½ cup cheese. Repeat the layers. Top the salad with avocado. To serve, pass salad around table followed by the dressing.

Brenda's Tips: This is a good way to introduce the family to a healthier diet. Try this for a Sunday lunch. At 17 grams of fiber per serving, this one dish is half your fiber for the day.

Nutrition Facts: Serving size, 1/6 recipe—calories 324, fiber 17 g, protein 15 g, fat 11 g, saturated fat 2 g, carbohydrate 45 g, cholesterol 0 mg, sodium 75 mg, sugars 3 g.

CRAB AND WHITE BEAN SALAD

serves four (4g fiber/serving)

- ⅓ cup chopped yellow pepper
- ¼ cup chopped red onion
- ¼ cup chopped celery
- 1 tablespoon white wine vinegar
- ½ tablespoon fresh lime juice
- ½ tablespoon olive oil
- Dash of hot sauce
- One 6-ounce can lump crabmeat, drained
- 1 cup cannellini beans (low-sodium), drained and rinsed
- 3 cups chopped salad greens

Combine all ingredients except greens; toss gently. Cover and chill. Serve over greens.

Brenda's Tips: The longer you let the beans chill in the refrigerator, the more flavorful this recipe becomes.

Nutrition Facts: Serving size, ¼ recipe—calories 122, fiber 4 g, protein 12 g, fat 3 g, saturated fat 0 g, carbohydrate 13 g, cholesterol 33 mg, sodium 134 mg, sugars 1 g.

MIXED SALAD WITH CHICKEN, FRUIT, AND NUTS

serves four (5g fiber/serving)

- 4 cups cooked chicken, torn into bite-size pieces
- ¼ cup minced red onion
- ¼ cup chopped pecans
- ¼ cup raw almonds, slivered*
- ¼ cup apple, chopped
- ¼ cup dried cherries
- ¼ cup carrots, julienned
- 1 teaspoon sesame seeds
- 1 kiwi, cut into ¼-inch rounds
- ¼ cup mango, sliced thin
- 2 teaspoons each of balsamic vinegar and olive oil

Combine everything except the kiwi, mango, vinegar, and oil. Make a bed of kiwi slices and put the salad on this. Garnish with mango. Drizzle with balsamic vinegar and olive oil.

Note: The sugars in this recipe are derived from fruit. To reduce the amount of sugar, use fresh cherries instead of dried.

Brenda's Tips: Because of the higher calories, I use this recipe as a meal—not as a side salad.

Nutrition Facts: Serving size, ¼ recipe—calories 458, fiber 5 g, protein 46 g, fat 17 g, saturated fat 2 g, carbohydrate 33 g, cholesterol 119 mg, sodium 117 mg, sugars 23 g.

SEAFOOD, SPINACH, AND ORANGE SALAD

serves four (6g fiber/serving)

- 12 cups baby spinach leaves, stems removed, loosely packed

- 3 navel oranges, halved

- 1 large red or yellow bell pepper

- 12 ounces cooked shrimp or fresh lump crabmeat

- 8 very thin slices of red onion

- 1 cup freshly squeezed orange juice

- Juice of 1 lime

- ¼ teaspoon turmeric

- 1 teaspoon marjoram

- 1½ tablespoons olive oil

- Freshly ground black pepper

- 1 lime cut into quarters (optional)

Divide the spinach among four dinner plates. On top of the spinach, arrange the oranges and bell pepper. On top of that arrange the shrimp or crab. Separate onions into rings and arrange over shrimp or crab.

In small bowl, swish together orange juice, lime juice, turmeric, marjoram, and olive oil; season to taste with fresh pepper. Spoon the dressing over each salad. Salads can be garnished with fresh lime quarters.

Brenda's Tips: Because of its vibrant color this is a great salad when you want to impress friends at a luncheon, and it tastes as good as it looks!

Nutrition Facts: Serving size, ¼ recipe—calories 245, fiber 6 g, protein 20 g, fat 7 g, saturated fat 1 g, carbohydrate 29 g, cholesterol 67 mg, sodium 327 mg, sugars 18 g.

SOUP AND STEW RECIPES

RED LENTIL SOUP

serves four to six (11g fiber/serving)

- 3 tablespoons olive oil
- ½ cup red onion
- ½ cup green pepper, chopped
- ½ cup red pepper, chopped
- 3 jalapeños
- 6 cloves garlic
- 2 cups dried red lentils, soaked overnight and rinsed
- 3 medium tomatoes, diced
- 4 ribs celery
- 4 cups reduced-sodium chicken stock
- 4 cups water
- 1 sprig of fresh marjoram

Put into a 4-quart pan at medium heat the oil, onion, peppers, jalapeños, and garlic. Sauté until onion turns translucent. Add lentils, tomatoes, celery, stock, and water; bring to a boil for 2 minutes. Cover and simmer for 20 minutes or until lentils are slightly crunchy. In either a traditional or a hand-wand-style blender, blend mixture on a low speed but allow some chunkiness to remain. Garnish with marjoram and serve with a side of nutty grain bread.

Brenda's Tips: This spicy lentil soup will warm up your day. It is great served with a flat bread such as lavosh.

Nutrition Facts: Serving size, 1 cup—calories 388, fiber 11 g, protein 23 g, fat 10 g, saturated fat 1 g, carbohydrate 55 g, cholesterol 0 mg, sodium 467 mg, sugars 5 g.

BUTTERNUT SQUASH SOUP

serves four (5g fiber/serving)

- 1 tablespoon olive oil
- 2 cups chopped onion
- ½ teaspoon ground nutmeg
- 4 cups cubed peeled butternut squash
- 1 apple (cored and peeled)
- 1½ cups low-sodium chicken stock
- 1 teaspoon sea salt
- ¼ cup plain yogurt

Heat oil in a large saucepan over medium heat. Add onion and nutmeg; sauté 6 minutes or until tender. Add squash cubes and apple, and cook 2 minutes, stirring frequently. Add stock and sea salt, bring to boil, reduce heat, and simmer 30 minutes until squash and apple are tender.

Place squash mixture in a blender or food processor and blend until smooth. Return squash mixture to pan, and cook until thoroughly heated. Ladle into bowls and top with yogurt.

Brenda's Tips: This is a very satisfying and filling soup. It's really good with a large salad!

Nutrition Facts: Serving size, 1 cup—calories 159, fiber 5 g, protein 4 g, fat 4 g, saturated fat 1 g, carbohydrate 30 g, cholesterol 2 mg, sodium 29 mg, sugars 12 g.

BLACK BEAN SOUP

serves four (21g fiber/serving)

- 1 tablespoon olive oil
- ½ cup diced celery
- ½ cup minced onion
- ¼ cup chopped green bell pepper
- 3 cloves garlic, minced
- 1½ teaspoons ground cumin
- 1 teaspoon dried oregano
- 1 teaspoon chili powder
- 1 teaspoon fresh black pepper
- 2 cups (low-sodium) chicken broth (may also use vegetable broth)
- 1 cup water
- Three 15-ounce cans low-sodium (or no-salt) black beans, rinsed and drained
- One 15-ounce can low-sodium stewed or diced tomatoes

Heat oil in medium stockpot over medium heat. Add celery, minced onion, and bell pepper. Cook about 10 minutes until tender. Add garlic and next 4 ingredients; cook 3 more minutes. Add broth, water, beans, and tomatoes. Bring to a boil, reduce heat, and simmer 15–30 minutes.

Brenda's Tips: This soup is very high in fiber! Did you know that one can of black beans has 19.4 grams of fiber!

Nutrition Facts: Serving size, 1 cup—calories 345, fiber 21 g, protein 22 g, fat 4 g, saturated fat 1 g, carbohydrate 59 g, cholesterol 0 mg, sodium 799 mg, sugars 1 g.

CHICKEN AND BEAN TORTILLA SOUP

serves eight (3g fiber/serving)

- 1 teaspoon olive oil
- 1 cup chopped onion
- 2 garlic cloves, minced
- 2 cups cooked, shredded chicken breast (skin removed)
- 1 cup low-sodium pinto beans
- 1 tablespoon chopped seeded jalapeño pepper
- 1 teaspoon ground cumin
- 1 teaspoon Worcestershire sauce
- ½ teaspoon chili powder
- Two 14-ounce cans low-sodium chicken broth
- One 14½-ounce can low-sodium diced peeled tomatoes
- 1¼ cups crushed, baked tortilla chips (about 16 chips)
- ½ cup plain low-fat yogurt (for garnish)

Heat oil in a Dutch oven over medium-high heat. Add onion and garlic; sauté 2 minutes. Stir in chicken and all remaining ingredients except tortilla chips and yogurt. Reduce heat; simmer 1 hour. Ladle soup into bowls; top with crushed tortilla chips and a dollop of yogurt.

Brenda's Tips: This is a good way of having Mexican food without the fat!

Nutrition Facts: Serving size, 1 cup—calories 233, fiber 3 g, protein 19 g, fat 3 g, saturated fat 1 g, carbohydrate 32 g, cholesterol 34 mg, sodium 392 mg, sugars 2 g.

WHITE BEAN STEW

serves four (15g fiber/serving)

- 2 cups chicken or vegetable stock (low-sodium)

- 3 cups purified water

- 2 tablespoons extra-virgin olive oil

- 1 large onion (peeled and cut into ½-inch pieces)

- 2 medium carrots (peeled and cut into ½-inch pieces)

- 1 large rib celery (cut into ½-inch pieces)

- Two 15-ounce cans low- or no-salt great northern beans

- 2½ cups chopped fresh kale

- Sea salt and pepper to taste

In a large pot, combine stock, water, olive oil, and onion. Simmer over medium heat 15 minutes. Then add carrots and celery. Cover and cook 10–15 minutes. Drain beans and stir into soup. Let simmer 5–10 more minutes. Add chopped greens. Season with salt and pepper. When greens become tender, the soup is done!

Brenda's Tips: This soup is very high in fiber and protein. It makes a complete meal, or serve it with a salad.

Nutrition Facts: Serving size, 1½ cups—calories 324, fiber 15 g, protein 18 g, fat 8 g, saturated fat 1 g, carbohydrate 48 g, cholesterol 0 mg, sodium 331 mg, sugars 4 g.

VEGETABLE BEAN CHILI

serves six (14g fiber/serving)

- 2 tablespoons olive oil

- 1 large onion

- 3 garlic cloves, crushed

- 3 cans diced tomatoes in juice

- One 4-ounce can mild green chilis

- ½ fresh jalapeño chili,
  seeded and chopped fine

- 2 to 3 tablespoons chili powder

- 1 tablespoon cumin

- 1 tablespoon dried chives

- 1 bay leaf

- One 15-ounce can red kidney
  beans (drained and rinsed)

- One 15-ounce can black or white
  kidney beans (drained and rinsed)

- 1 large green bell pepper
  (cut into ½-inch pieces)

- 1 large red bell pepper (cut
  into ½-inch pieces)

- 2 ears of fresh corn
  (or 1 cup frozen)

- Sea salt and pepper to taste

- ¼ cup chopped fresh cilantro
  leaves (loosely packed)

In a large heavy pot, heat olive oil over medium-high heat. Add onion and garlic and sauté, stirring often, for about 5 minutes, until the onion is translucent.

Add tomatoes (with juice), chilis, jalapeño, chili powder, cumin, chives, and bay leaf. Cook over medium heat 10 minutes. Add beans, bell peppers, and corn. Bring to a boil: reduce heat to medium-low; and simmer about 35 minutes, stirring occasionally, until chili is thick. Season to taste with the sea salt and pepper. Stir in cilantro. Remove bay leaf before serving.

Note: You can use low-sodium or no-salt-added canned vegetables.

Brenda's Tips: I start with 2 tablespoons of chili powder and, at the end of cooking, taste it to see if it has enough heat. If not, I add the other tablespoon of chili powder. This recipe can be frozen in individual servings for later use.

Nutrition Facts: Serving size, 1 cup—calories 258, fiber 14 g, protein 12 g, fat 5 g, saturated fat 1 g, carbohydrate 46 g, cholesterol 0 mg, sodium 614 mg, sugar 2 g.

VEGETABLE SOUP

serves eight (4g fiber/serving)

- 2 tablespoons extra-virgin olive oil
- 2 cups chopped onion
- 5 cloves garlic, minced
- 2 ribs celery, chopped
- 1 cup green beans, cut into 2-inch pieces
- ½ cup carrots, cut into ¼-inch pieces
- 1 medium zucchini (halved lengthwise and sliced)
- 5 fresh basil leaves
- 1 teaspoon oregano
- 1 teaspoon rosemary
- 4 cups low-sodium vegetable broth
- 4 cups purified water
- One 15-ounce can low-sodium light kidney beans (drained)
- 4 cups chopped and seeded tomato
- 2 cups shredded green cabbage
- 1 teaspoon sea salt
- 1 teaspoon fresh ground black pepper

Heat oil in a stockpot over medium-high heat. Add onion and garlic and sauté 2 minutes. Stir in celery and next 10 ingredients. Bring to a boil and simmer 30 minutes. Add cabbage, salt, and pepper; cook 5 minutes until cabbage wilts. Serve.

Brenda's Tips: You can increase the fiber content in this recipe by adding table fiber. This soup is so low in calories that it could be used as one of the snacks.

Nutrition Facts: Serving size, 1 cup—calories 87, fiber 4 g, protein 2 g, fat 0 g, saturated fat 0 g, carbohydrate 12 g, cholesterol 0 mg, sodium 387 mg, sugars 7 g.

TOMATO BASIL SOUP

serves eight (2g fiber/serving)

- 4 cups chopped seeded peeled tomato
- 4 cups low-sodium tomato juice
- ⅓ cup fresh basil leaves
- 1 cup low-sodium chicken stock
- ¼ teaspoon sea salt
- ¼ teaspoon pepper
- ½ cup plain low-fat yogurt

Bring tomato and juice to a boil in a large saucepan. Reduce heat. Simmer uncovered 30 minutes.

Place tomato mixture and basil (leaving a few fresh leaves for garnish) in a blender or food processor; process until smooth. Return pureed mixture to pan; add chicken stock, sea salt, and pepper. Add yogurt, stirring with a whisk. Cook over medium heat until thick (about 5 minutes). Serve soup with additional fresh basil leaves.

Brenda's Tips: This soup can also be used as a snack in either Phase One or Phase Two, even with a slice of whole-grain bread or some flax crackers. Sprinkle with table fiber to boost fiber content.

Nutrition Facts: Serving size, 1 cup—calories 49, fiber 2 g, protein 3 g, fat 0 g, saturated fat 0 g, carbohydrate 10 g, cholesterol 1 mg, sodium 717 mg, sugars 8 g.

MEAL RECIPES

Following are five recipes for complete meals. You should not have to add any more items to these, as they all contain protein, vegetables, and complex carbohydrates.

BEEF AND VEGETABLE FRIED RICE

serves two (4g fiber/serving)

- 2 tablespoons peanut oil
- ¼ pound beef, any cut, sliced into thin strips
- 1 rib celery, cut lengthwise
- ¼ cup bean sprouts
- 12 snow peas
- ¼ cup cremini* mushrooms
- 5 broccoli florets
- ¼ cup carrots, julienned
- 1 radish, sliced
- 1 teaspoon ginger, grated
- 2 cloves garlic, chopped
- 1 cup brown rice, cooked
- 2 teaspoons low-sodium soy sauce
- ½ teaspoon sesame seed oil
- 1 egg, beaten
- 1 teaspoon sesame seeds

Put into a large skillet or wok, at high heat, 1 tablespoon peanut oil and the beef. Sauté beef until done. Set beef aside. Add remaining peanut oil and all vegetables, ginger, and garlic and stir frequently for about 3–4 minutes or until vegetables are tender-crisp. Add rice, soy sauce, and sesame oil and stir frequently to keep rice from sticking. Remove from heat and add cooked beef. Place in serving bowl or plate. Return pan to medium heat and cook egg quickly, whisking with fork. Add cooked egg to beef mixture. Garnish with sesame seeds.

*Note: * A dark brown mushroom with a round cap*

Brenda's Tips: This makes a great weekend lunch for two. For a lighter meal, try using chicken or make it vegetarian.

Nutrition Facts: Serving size, ½ recipe—calories 437, fiber 4 g, protein 20 g, fat 26 g, saturated fat 6 g, carbohydrate 32 g, cholesterol 120 mg, sodium 275 mg, sugars 3 g.

WEST INDIES WILD SALMON WITH BROWN RICE

serves two (5g fiber / serving)

RICE

- ½ cup short-grain brown rice
- 1 teaspoon butter
- ¼ cup fresh basil leaves cut into thin strips
- ¼ cup pineapple, chopped and drained

WET RUB

- 1 teaspoon soy sauce
- ½ teaspoon honey
- ½ teaspoon fresh grated ginger
- ½ teaspoon crushed red pepper
- ½ teaspoon blackstrap molasses
- 1 tablespoon olive oil
- Drizzle of toasted sesame oil
- Pinch of salt
- 1 teaspoon fresh ground black pepper

FISH

- Two 3-ounce wild salmon fillets
- 1 tablespoon olive oil
- ¼ cup chives, finely chopped

Put rice into 1 cup boiling water. Reduce to simmer. Cover and cook approximately 20–30 minutes or until all water is absorbed and rice is tender. Remove from heat; gently stir in butter, basil, and pineapple. Then cover and set aside.

Preheat oven to 375°F.

In a small bowl, combine all wet-rub ingredients except black pepper.

Wash salmon and pat dry.

Glaze the top of the fish with the wet rub liberally, then dust with black pepper. Heat olive oil in skillet on medium-high heat. Place salmon, skin side down, in skillet for approximately 3–4 minutes or until skin turns crisp. Then place entire skillet in oven for another 6–8 minutes or until the salmon reaches the desired doneness.

Plate rice with salmon and garnish with chives.

Brenda's Tips: Salmon is a great way to get your omega-3 fatty acids, and it's delicious, too!

Nutrition Facts: Serving size, ½ recipe—calories 469, fiber 5 g, protein 26 g, fat 25 g, saturated fat 4 g, carbohydrate 36 g, cholesterol 65 mg, sodium 283 mg, sugars 8 g.

VEGETABLE LASAGNA

serves eight (4g fiber/serving)

- 1 pound rice lasagna noodles
- Pump or spray olive oil
- 2 cups kale, chopped
- 3 cups shredded mozzarella
- 1 medium carrot, sliced in strips
- 1 medium Spanish onion, chopped fine
- 10 asparagus spears, cut into ¼-inch pieces
- 1 red pepper, chopped
- ½ cup freshly grated Parmesan

CHEESE MIXTURE
- 1 cup low-fat ricotta cheese
- 1 cup plain yogurt
- ½ cup parsley
- Red pepper flakes
- Salt and pepper to taste

Bring pot of lightly salted water to a boil and cook pasta. Remove from water and drain. Lay the sheets of pasta flat in layers of plastic wrap or waxed paper until ready to build lasagna. Preheat oven to 400°F. Spray bottom of 6-inch baking dish with olive oil.

Combine ricotta cheese, yogurt, parsley, red pepper flakes, salt and pepper in mixing bowl. Set aside.

Build lasagna from bottom up in baking dish. Start with the pasta; add kale, ricotta cheese mixture, and 1 cup mozzarella; and top with pasta. Add second layer of carrot, onion, ricotta cheese mixture, and 1 cup mozzarella, and top with pasta. Add third layer, consisting of asparagus, red pepper, ricotta cheese mixture, 1 cup mozzarella, and pasta. Sprinkle top with Parmesan cheese. Bake in preheated oven for 1 hour.

Brenda's Tips: This is a great make-ahead dish to be used throughout the week or to freeze and use when you do not have time to cook.

Nutrition Facts: Serving size, ⅛ recipe—calories 483, fiber 4 g, protein 23 g, fat 15 g, saturated fat 9 g, carbohydrate 59 g, cholesterol 52 mg, sodium 589 mg, sugars 3 g.

TURKEY ROLL WITH GOAT CHEESE AND SPINACH

serves four (3g fiber/serving)

- 1-pound turkey breast, pounded to cutlet

- 1 sweet potato, peeled and sliced thin

- 1 cup whole-leaf fresh spinach

- ¼ cup frozen unsweetened cherries

- ¼ cup pecans, chopped

- 2 cloves garlic, minced

- ¼ cup goat cheese

- 2 tablespoons rice flour

- Spray or pump olive oil

- Salt and pepper to taste

Preheat oven to 375°F.

Lay turkey breast on cutting board or firm surface. Cover with plastic wrap or waxed paper and pound very thin with a flat meat mallet and salt lightly. Layer thin sweet potato slices, spinach, cherries, pecans, garlic, and goat cheese onto cutlet. Roll tightly, tie with string, and dust with rice flour. Spray skillet with olive oil, heat to medium, add the turkey roll and brown on all sides. Place covered skillet in oven and bake for 30–45 minutes or until cooked through. Remove from heat and allow to rest for 10 minutes before slicing. May be served plain or with your choice of vegetables.

Brenda's Tips: You can substitute any of your favorite vegetables or even fruit. Try making several rolls with different stuffing ingredients for a party.

Nutrition Facts: Serving size, ¼ pound—calories 396, fiber 3 g, protein 36 g, fat 18 g, saturated fat 5 g, carbohydrate 20 g, cholesterol 99 mg, sodium 185 mg, sugars 3 g.

PISTACHIO-CRUSTED CHICKEN WITH SMASHED SWEET POTATOES

serves two (8g fiber/serving)

CHICKEN
- 1 chicken breast
- ¼ cup rice flour
- 1 egg and ¼ cup water, beaten
- ¼ cup raw pistachios, chopped fine
- Pump or spray olive oil

SMASHED SWEET POTATOES
- Two 5-inch-long sweet potatoes, peeled and cubed
- ½ orange, zested and juiced
- ½ cup reduced-sodium chicken broth
- ¼ teaspoon grated nutmeg
- Salt and pepper to taste

SAUTÉED COLLARD GREENS
- 2 cups collard greens, confetti-cut
- ½ cup water
- 1 tablespoon olive oil

Fillet chicken breast into two cutlets on cutting board. Lay plastic wrap or waxed paper over chicken and pound to ¼ inch with flat meat mallet. Salt slightly. Preheat oven to 350°F. Coat chicken with rice flour and then dredge in egg batter. Place in small bowl and cover with pistachios. Spray skillet with olive oil; heat to medium. Sauté both sides of chicken approximately 4–5 minutes each until golden brown. Place skillet in preheated oven for an additional 10–15 minutes.

Boil sweet potatoes for approximately 10–15 minutes or until tender but not too soft; then drain. In a large bowl, combine potatoes, orange zest and juice, chicken broth, nutmeg, and salt and pepper. Mash. Over medium heat, sauté collard greens with water, stirring frequently, for approximately 6–8 minutes. Cover for 1 minute, allowing greens to steam. Drizzle olive oil over greens.

On each plate, layer half the sweet potatoes and half the greens and place a chicken cutlet on top.

Nutrition Facts: Serving size, ½ cutlet—calories 456, fiber 8 g, protein 26 g, fat 17 g, saturated fat 3 g, carbohydrate 51 g, cholesterol 127 mg, sodium 344 mg, sugars 10 g.

POULTRY RECIPES

SEARED CHICKEN WITH GREENS, RASPBERRIES, AND PEAR

serves two (6g fiber/serving)

- ⅛ cup balsamic vinegar
- 2 tablespoons freshly squeezed lime juice
- 1 garlic clove, crushed
- 1 tablespoon dried thyme
- 1 small red chili, chopped
- 2 breasts of chicken
- Spray oil
- 1 tablespoon extra-virgin olive oil
- 1 teaspoon Dijon mustard
- Salt and pepper to taste
- 2½ cups spinach
- 1 pear, cored and cubed
- ½ cup raw raspberries

For the marinade: Mix 1 tablespoon of the vinegar, the lime juice, and the crushed garlic with half of the thyme and chopped chili in a bowl. Pour marinade and chicken into large ziplock bag and refrigerate for at least 2 hours. When ready to use, remove chicken and discard remaining marinade.

Preheat oven to 350° F. On stovetop, heat ovenproof frying pan to medium, coat pan with spray oil, and sear chicken for 3 minutes on each side. Place pan in oven until chicken is cooked throughout. Allow chicken to rest, then slice diagonally.

Combine olive oil, remaining vinegar and thyme, mustard, salt, and pepper, and mix well. Toss in spinach and pear. Plate greens, top with chicken, and finish with a sprinkle of raspberries.

Brenda's Tips: This recipe makes a great dinner—prepare and marinate the chicken in the morning, and serve it with brown rice. It also makes a great lunch served just with the greens and fruit.

Nutrition Facts: Serving size, 1 breast—calories 299, fiber 6 g, protein 30 g, fat 9 g, saturated fat 1 g, carbohydrate 26 g, cholesterol 68 mg, sodium 175 mg, sugars 14 g.

GRILLED CHICKEN KEBABS

serves four (1g fiber/serving)

- 3 chicken breasts, cut into large cubes
- 12 cherry tomatoes
- 6 large mushrooms, halved
- 1 clove garlic, crushed
- Zest of ½ lemon
- 1 tablespoon fresh lemon juice
- 1 tablespoon olive oil
- ½ tablespoon fresh oregano leaves, chopped

Soak four wooden skewers for 30 minutes to prevent burning, or use four metal skewers. Alternate chicken, tomato, and mushroom on skewers. Repeat until skewers are full. Combine garlic, lemon zest, lemon juice, olive oil, and chopped oregano in a bowl. Put skewers into a large dish and pour marinade over them, lightly turning to coat. Marinate for 2 hours or overnight.

Place chicken on heated grill and cook until chicken is done, turning occasionally. Serve with salad.

Brenda's Tips: These kebabs are a great, easy way to enjoy grilling.

Nutrition Facts: Serving size, 1 kebab—calories 147, fiber 1 g, protein 22 g, fat 5 g, saturated fat 1 g, carbohydrate 4 g, cholesterol 51 mg, sodium 62 mg, sugars 2 g.

ZESTY CHICKEN PATTIES

serves two (1g fiber/serving)

- ½ pound ground chicken
- 2 shallots, chopped
- 2 tablespoons chopped coriander
- 1 clove garlic, minced
- ½ teaspoon cayenne pepper
- 1 egg white, lightly beaten
- Salt and pepper to taste
- ½ tablespoon olive oil
- 1 lemon, halved

Mix together all ingredients except oil and lemon. Shape mixture into two patties and chill for 30 minutes to let set. Heat oil in pan and cook patties over medium heat on each side until done. Squeeze lemon over cooked patties and serve with green salad.

Brenda's Tips: You can use this recipe with any ground meat of your choosing. It's great with ground turkey!

Nutrition Facts: Serving size, 1 patty—calories 272, fiber 1 g, protein 23 g, fat 18 g, saturated fat 1 g, carbohydrate 6 g, cholesterol 93 mg, sodium 175 mg, sugars 1 g.

ASIAN CHICKEN WITH BOK CHOY

serves two (2g fiber/serving)

- 1 tablespoon low-sodium soy sauce

- 1 tablespoon rice wine vinegar

- ½ teaspoon sesame oil

- ½ tablespoon fresh grated ginger

- 2 chicken breasts

- ½ pound bok choy, cleaned and ends removed

- 5 dried shiitake mushrooms

- ¼ cup low-sodium chicken stock

- ½ tablespoon arrowroot flour or cornstarch

Combine soy sauce, vinegar, sesame oil and grated ginger in bowl. Pour this marinade and the chicken into a ziplock bag, shake to cover, and marinate for at least 2 hours. When ready to cook, remove chicken and reserve marinade.

Put chicken in bamboo steamer basket over boiling water in medium saucepan. Cover and let steam for 6 minutes; turn chicken over and steam for an additional 6 minutes. Place bok choy on top of chicken and continue steaming until chicken is done and bok choy is tender. Place reserved marinade and mushrooms in saucepan over medium heat. Simmer until mushrooms are tender.

In separate bowl, add enough of the chicken stock to arrowroot flour or cornstarch to make a paste. Add the paste and remaining stock to mushroom marinade and continue simmering until sauce thickens. Plate bok choy and chicken and add sauce to taste.

Brenda's Tips: To up the fiber content, serve this Asian meal with brown rice.

Nutrition Facts: Serving size, 1 breast—calories 199, fiber 2 g, protein 30 g, fat 3 g, saturated fat 1 g, carbohydrate 13 g, cholesterol 68 mg, sodium 511 mg, sugars 0 g.

CHICKEN IN A LETTUCE BOWL

serves two (1g fiber/serving)

- 1 tablespoon olive oil
- 8 ounces minced (or ground) chicken
- 1 clove garlic
- ½ can water chestnuts, chopped
- ½ tablespoon oyster sauce
- 1½ teaspoons low-sodium soy sauce
- 2 spring onions
- 2 whole lettuce leaves

Heat large wok or large frying pan over high heat; add oil; and swirl oil to coat pan. Add minced chicken and garlic and stir-fry for 3–4 minutes or until the chicken is cooked through. Keep mixture loose. Pour off excess liquid. Turn down heat and add water chestnuts, oyster sauce, soy sauce, and onions.

Trim lettuce leaves to form two lettuce cups. Divide mixture into them.

Brenda's Tips: This may be served with brown rice. You could also use sprinkle table fiber to up the fiber content.

Nutrition Facts: Serving size, 1 stuffed leaf—calories 212, fiber 1 g, protein 27 g, fat 8 g, saturated fat 1 g, carbohydrate 6 g, cholesterol 66 mg, sodium 333 mg, sugars 1 g.

CHICKEN MARSALA

serves two (1g fiber/serving)

- 2 boneless, skinless chicken breasts
- 1 tablespoon rice flour
- ¼ teaspoon salt
- ¼ teaspoon pepper
- ½ tablespoon olive oil
- ¼ cup presliced mushrooms
- ¼ cup marsala wine
- ¼ cup fat-free, low-sodium chicken broth
- 1 tablespoon fresh lemon juice
- ½ tablespoon chopped curly Italian parsley

Pound chicken between 2 pieces of plastic wrap or waxed paper to about ½-inch thick, using a meat mallet or rolling pin. Mix flour, salt, and pepper. Dredge chicken in flour mixture. Shake off excess.

Heat oil in a large skillet over medium-high heat. Add chicken and brown on each side for about 3 minutes. Remove chicken and set aside. Add mushrooms, wine, broth, and juice and simmer 10 minutes or until mixture is reduced to 2/3 cup. Return chicken to pan, turning to coat well. Cover and cook 5 minutes until chicken is done. Sprinkle with parsley.

Brenda's Tips: You can use spinkle table fiber to up the fiber. This is really good served with long-grain brown rice and a side salad.

Nutrition Facts: Serving size, 1 breast—calories 269, fiber 1 g, protein 29 g, fat 5 g, saturated fat 1 g, carbohydrate 14 g, cholesterol 68 mg, sodium 441 mg, sugars 1 g.

CHICKEN PICCATA

serves two (1g fiber/serving)

- 2 chicken breasts, skin removed
- ¼ cup rice flour
- ¼ teaspoon salt
- ¼ teaspoon pepper
- 1 teaspoon olive oil
- ¾ cup dry white wine
- 1 tablespoon fresh lemon juice
- 1 tablespoon capers
- ¼ cup chopped flat-leaf parsley

Place chicken breast between 2 sheets of plastic wrap or waxed paper and flatten to ¼-inch thickness, using a mallet. Combine flour, salt, and pepper; dredge chicken in flour mixture. Heat olive oil in skillet over medium-high heat. Add chicken; cook 3 minutes on each side until browned. Add half of the wine, the juice, and the capers to pan, scraping pan to loosen brown bits. Cook 2 minutes; remove chicken from the pan; keep warm. Stir in rest of wine and cook until it is reduced by half. Stir in fresh chopped parsley.

Brenda's Tips: This is great served with long-grain brown rice and a small dinner salad.

Nutrition Facts: Serving size, 1 breast—calories 298, fiber 1 g, protein 29 g, fat 4 g, saturated fat 1 g, carbohydrate 19 g, cholesterol 68 mg, sodium 500 mg, sugars 1 g.

CHICKEN WRAPS

serves two (2g fiber/serving)

- 2 tablespoons hummus

- 3 ounces low-fat plain yogurt

- 1 spring onion, diced

- 1 chicken breast (cooked, no skin)

- Two 6-inch tortilla wraps
  (whole grain)

- 2 leaves of romaine lettuce

- ½ carrot, julienned

- ¼ cup red bell pepper, julienned

Mix hummus, yogurt, and onion. Cut chicken into cubes (about ½-inch pieces). Add chicken to mixture and stir well. Arrange tortilla and lettuce, add chicken mixture, then add carrot and pepper. Roll firmly and slice.

Brenda's Tips: This is a good recipe for leftover chicken. You can use mixable fiber for more fiber content.

Nutrition Facts: Serving size, 1 wrap—calories 305, fiber 2 g, protein 33 g, fat 7 g, saturated fat 2 g, carbohydrate 25 g, cholesterol 76 mg, sodium 292 mg, sugars 4 g.

CROCK-POT CHICKEN CACCIATORE

serves six (5g fiber/serving)

- 1 teaspoon onion powder
- 1 teaspoon garlic powder
- 1 teaspoon oregano
- 1 teaspoon basil
- ¾ teaspoon black pepper (freshly ground)
- 3 chicken breasts (halved, boned, skinned)
- 3 chicken thighs (halved, boned, skinned)
- 1 tablespoon olive oil
- 2 cups sliced mushrooms
- 1½ cups red bell pepper strips
- 1½ cups green bell pepper strips
- 1 cup thin-sliced onion
- One 28-ounce can no-salt-added tomatoes
- One 6-ounce can tomato paste, low-sodium
- 2 bay leaves
- 1 tablespoon balsamic vinegar

Mix first five ingredients. Dredge chicken in these spices. Set aside. Put 1 tablespoon olive oil in bottom of Crock-Pot. Add mushrooms, peppers, and onion. Add tomatoes, tomato paste, bay leaves, and vinegar. Add spiced chicken and any remaining spice mixture. Cook on low 7–9 hours. Serve with brown rice pasta and a salad.

Brenda's Tips: This dish is for a crowd. It's healthy, but no one will ever know!

Nutrition Facts: Serving size, 1 breast or thigh—calories 197, fiber 5 g, protein 22 g, fat 4 g, saturated fat 1 g, carbohydrate 20 g, cholesterol 51 mg, sodium 108 mg, sugars 11 g.

LEMON CHICKEN

serves two (2g fiber/serving)

- 2 boneless, skinless chicken breasts

- 1 egg white

- 2 tablespoons rice flour

- 1 tablespoon freshly grated Parmesan cheese

- 1 tablespoon chopped Italian parsley

- Dash of salt and pepper

- 1 teaspoon olive oil

- Juice of ½ lemon

- ¼ cup white wine or chicken stock

Preheat oven to 450°F. Place chicken between sheets of plastic wrap or waxed paper and pound with smooth side of meat mallet. This helps to tenderize the chicken; ½ inch in thickness is fine. Set aside.

Lightly beat egg white in a medium-size bowl. Add rice flour, Parmesan, parsley, salt, and pepper. Coat chicken evenly.

Heat oil in a medium-size ovenproof skillet. Brown chicken (3 minutes) on each side. Remove chicken and set aside. Add the juice of ½ lemon and wine to pan, making sure to incorporate the bits in the pan with the liquids. Let this reduce slightly, add back the chicken, and bake for 20 minutes.

Brenda's Tips: This dish is so good with some greens, like kale or collards, sautéed in a pan.

Nutrition Facts: Serving size, 1 breast—calories 357, fiber 2 g, protein 44 g, fat 5 g, saturated fat 1 g, carbohydrate 25 g, cholesterol 71 mg, sodium 372 mg, sugars 2 g.

TURKEY BURGERS

serves two (1g fiber/serving)

- ½ pound ground turkey breast
- 1 clove garlic, minced
- ½ teaspoon Cajun seasoning
- Dash of black pepper
- 2 tablespoons light teriyaki sauce
- Cooking spray
- 1 medium onion, sliced ¼ inch thick
- 1 teaspoon olive oil

Combine first five ingredients in a large bowl. Divide mixture into two patties. Put cooking spray in pan and place over medium heat. Add onion slices and cook until they are tender and brown. Remove onion from pan and set aside. Add olive oil to pan and add patties. Cook 5–10 minutes over medium heat, turning to brown both sides when patties are done. Plate turkey patty with onion on top.

Brenda's Tips: This would be good with a large green salad, or sautéed vegetables. Also, you could add mixable fiber to the turkey patty to up the fiber content.

Nutrition Facts: Serving size, 1 burger—calories 227, fiber 1 g, protein 21 g, fat 12 g, saturated fat 3 g, carbohydrate 8 g, cholesterol 90 mg, sodium 369 mg, sugars 4 g.

ZESTY LEMON HERB TURKEY BREAST

serves eight (0g fiber/serving)

- Juice and zest of 2 lemons
- 2 tablespoons fresh rosemary
- 1 teaspoon sage
- 2 tablespoons Dijon mustard
- ½ cup water
- 2 cloves (crushed) garlic
- Salt and pepper to taste
- 1 boneless turkey breast, about 2 pounds

Mix all ingredients except turkey to make the marinade. Place turkey breast and marinade in a large plastic bag. Place in a large bowl. Make sure all the turkey is coated. Refrigerate 4–6 hours or overnight.

Place turkey and marinade in a Crock-Pot. Cover and cook on low for 8 hours or until tender.

Brenda's Tips: This will serve eight people, or you can use the leftover turkey for a sandwich later.

Nutrition Facts: Serving size, ¼ pound—calories 133, fiber 0 g, protein 28 g, fat 1 g, saturated fat 1 g, carbohydrate 2 g, cholesterol 71 mg, sodium 367 mg, sugars 0 g.

CHICKEN ASPARAGUS STIR-FRY

serves two (5g fiber/serving)

- 1 tablespoon olive oil
- 1 garlic clove, crushed
- 1 tablespoon sliced fresh ginger
- One 8-ounce chicken breast, sliced
- 1 shallot
- 3 ounces fresh asparagus (sliced on the diagonal)
- 2 tablespoons low-sodium soy sauce
- ¼ cup water
- 2 ounces slivered almonds (roasted)

Heat large frying pan over high heat. Add oil and swirl to coat. Add garlic, ginger, and chicken. Stir-fry 1–2 minutes, until chicken turns color. Add shallot and asparagus and stir-fry for 2 more minutes. Reduce heat and simmer for 2 minutes. Stir in soy sauce and ¼ cup water. Cover and continue to simmer for 2 more minutes. Cook until chicken and vegetables are tender. Toss in almonds.

Brenda's Tips: This is a quick dinner recipe! It should be served with long-grain brown rice.

Nutrition Facts: Serving size, ½ recipe—calories 323, fiber 5 g, protein 22 g, fat 22 g, saturated fat 2 g, carbohydrate 12 g, cholesterol 34 mg, sodium 641 mg, sugars 3 g.

FISH RECIPES

BAKED FISH

serves two (4g fiber/serving)

- Two 4-ounce white fish fillets (flounder or tilapia)

- One 10-ounce package fresh spinach

- 2 small plum tomatoes, sliced

- 2 shallots, sliced thin

- 1 tablespoon chopped black olives

- 1 tablespoon capers

- 2 tablespoons fresh orange juice

- Pepper to taste

Preheat oven to 400°F. Place fillets in a shallow glass baking dish. Top fillets with spinach, tomatoes, shallots, olives, and capers. Drizzle orange juice over entire dish. Cook fish in oven about 10 minutes per inch of thickness. Sprinkle with pepper. Serve immediately.

Brenda's Tips: This recipe can be made with frozen spinach; but it will increase salt intake, even if the package says "no added salt."

Nutrition Facts: Serving size, 1 fillet—calories 168, fiber 4 g, protein 26 g, fat 3 g, saturated fat 1 g, carbohydrate 11 g, cholesterol 54 mg, sodium 457 mg, sugars 3 g.

GRILLED MAHIMAHI WITH SPINACH

serves two (2g fiber/serving)

- 2 mahimahi steaks
- 2 teaspoons olive oil
- 1 shallot
- 2 cloves garlic
- Sea salt and pepper to taste
- 2 large tomatoes, peeled, seeded, and chopped
- 2 cups spinach (washed)

Rinse steaks and pat dry. Brush with some of the olive oil and grill over medium-hot coals. Use remaining olive oil to coat bottom of a skillet. Sauté shallot, garlic, salt, and pepper until shallot is tender. Add tomatoes and spinach. Cook until spinach starts to wilt. Plate mixture and top with fish. Garnish with fresh lime juice.

Brenda's Tips: This recipe can be made with frozen spinach, but it will increase the salt intake, even if the package says "no added salt." You can also use mixable fiber in the vegetables to increase the fiber content of this dish.

Nutrition Facts: Serving size, 1 fillet—calories 188, fiber 2 g, protein 23 g, fat 5 g, saturated fat 1 g, carbohydrate 6 g, cholesterol 0 mg, sodium 108 mg, sugars 2 g.

GRILLED WILD SALMON WITH MANGO RELISH

serves two (1g fiber/serving)

MANGO RELISH

- ½ small mango (diced)

- 2 tablespoons red bell pepper (diced)

- 1 tablespoon red onion (diced)

- 1 tablespoon parsley (chopped fine)

- 1 tablespoon cilantro (chopped)

- 1 teaspoon lime zest

- ½ tablespoon garlic, minced

- 1 teaspoon lime juice

- Two 4-ounce wild salmon fillets

- Sea salt and pepper to taste

For relish, combine all relish ingredients and chill in refrigerator for 1 hour.

Season the fillets with the salt and pepper and grill on a hot grill 4 minutes on one side and 4 minutes on the other side. Cook until fish flakes.

Serve relish over fish.

Brenda's Tips: This relish is delicious with any fish. Also, this dish is recommended with my sweet potato mash and steamed spinach, recipes found later in this chapter.

Nutrition Facts: Serving size, 1 fillet—calories 209, fiber 1 g, protein 24 g, fat 7 g, saturated fat 1 g, carbohydrate 12 g, cholesterol 63 mg, sodium 56 mg, sugars 8 g.

WILD SALMON WITH CITRUS MARINADE

serves two (0g fiber/serving)

- ¼ cup balsamic vinegar
- ¼ cup fresh orange juice
- ¼ cup fresh lemon or lime juice
- 2 teaspoons spicy brown mustard
- Two 4-ounce wild salmon fillets

Combine vinegar, orange juice, lemon or lime juice, and mustard in a bowl. Whisk together with a fork. Add salmon and coat well to marinate. Place in refrigerator for 1–2 hours. Remove salmon from marinade and place on a hot grill for 2 minutes. Grill the flesh side first, then turn the salmon skin side down and use the marinade to baste while cooking. Cook 4–5 more minutes. If necessary, cover with aluminum pan to help cook completely. Cook until fish turns pale pink or flakes with a fork.

Brenda's Tips: To get your fiber content for this meal, serve the fish with ½ cup brown rice and 2 cups steamed spinach.

Nutrition Facts: Serving size, 1 fillet—calories 215, fiber 0 g, protein 23 g, fat 8 g, saturated fat 1 g, carbohydrate 11 g, cholesterol 63 mg, sodium 115 mg, sugars 8 g.

VEGETABLE RECIPES

Use these vegetable recipes with the poultry or fish recipes to complete the meal.

ROASTED BROCCOLI WITH LEMON AND SHALLOTS

serves two (2g fiber/serving)

- 2 cups broccoli
- ½ cup finely sliced shallots
- 1 teaspoon olive oil
- Sea salt and pepper to taste
- Juice of ½ small lemon

Preheat oven to 450°F. Toss broccoli with shallots, oil, salt, and pepper.

Place on a large baking sheet (with sides) and roast until broccoli is tender and brown on bottom, 10–12 minutes. Remove from oven and sprinkle with lemon juice. Toss gently and serve.

Brenda's Tips: Roasting broccoli is a very delicious alternative to steaming.

Nutrition Facts: Serving size, 1 cup—calories 95, fiber 2 g, protein 4 g, fat 3 g, saturated fat 0 g, carbohydrate 17 g, cholesterol 0 mg, sodium 37 mg, sugars 4 g.

CAULIFLOWER MASH

serves four (1g fiber/serving)

- 1 pound cauliflower, trimmed
- ½ cup water
- ½ cup Pacific Natural Foods low-sodium chicken broth
- 1 tablespoon olive oil

Cut cauliflower, including the core, into 1-inch pieces. Bring the water and stock to a boil in a large pot. Add cauliflower pieces. Cook until tender, 20–30 minutes. Drain cauliflower in colander and press with a small plate to release all the liquid in the cauliflower (this step is important for the texture of the dish). Transfer cauliflower into a food processor. Add olive oil and puree the mixture until it becomes smooth and creamy.

Brenda's Tips: This is a great substitute for mashed potatoes. You may add table fiber to up the fiber content.

Nutrition Facts: Serving size, ½ cup—calories 95, fiber 1 g, protein 2 g, fat 3 g, saturated fat 0 g, carbohydrate 4 g, cholesterol 0 mg, sodium 50 mg, sugars 2 g.

MEDLEY OF ROASTED VEGETABLES

serves four (5g fiber/serving)

- 1½ cups onions (cut into ½-inch pieces)

- 2 cups carrots (cut in ½-inch pieces)

- 6 ounces baby turnips, peeled and cut into ¼-inch wedges

- 6 ounces beets (cut into ¼-inch wedges)

- 1 tablespoon olive oil

- Sea salt and fresh black pepper to taste

- 10 sprigs of thyme

- 1 teaspoon lemon zest

- 2 tablespoons apple cider

- 2 tablespoons Italian parsley, finely chopped

Preheat oven to 450°F. Put vegetables into a large bowl and toss with oil, salt, pepper, thyme, lemon zest, and apple cider. Spread vegetables in a single layer on a baking sheet with sides. Roast, turning vegetables twice, until tender, about 30 minutes.

Transfer vegetables to a large serving dish. Sprinkle with parsley and serve.

Brenda's Tips: You can replace one of the vegetables above with any of your favorite root vegetables, like parsnips or leeks.

Nutrition Facts: Serving size, ¼ recipe—calories 113, fiber 5 g, protein 3 g, fat 4 g, saturated fat 1 g, carbohydrate 22 g, cholesterol 0 mg, sodium 119 mg, sugars 14 g.

SOUTHERN KALE

serves six (3g fiber/serving)

- 1 tablespoon olive oil
- 2 teaspoons minced garlic
- ½ cup low-sodium chicken stock
- 15 cups rinsed, stemmed, and torn kale
- ¼ teaspoon crushed red pepper
- Black pepper to taste

Heat oil in a deep skillet over medium heat. Add garlic and stock; stir. Add kale by handfuls, stirring to make room for more leaves. Cover with a lid and cook, stirring occasionally for 10–15 minutes. Uncover and cook until leaves are tender. Add red pepper and black pepper. Toss and serve.

Brenda's Tips: You can use collard greens instead of kale.

Nutrition Facts: Serving size, 1/6 recipe—calories 114, fiber 3 g, protein 6 g, fat 3 g, saturated fat 0 g, carbohydrate 17 g, cholesterol 0 mg, sodium 107 mg, sugars 0 g.

SPAGHETTI SQUASH

serves four (5g fiber/serving)

- 1 medium spaghetti squash

Preheat oven to 400°F. Cut squash in half lengthwise. Remove seeds. Place halves facedown in a baking dish; put about ½ inch of water in bottom of dish. Place dish in oven and bake 30 minutes or until tender. When cooled, turn squash over. Using the tongs of a fork, scrape the squash. It will begin to string like spaghetti.

Brenda's Tips: This is a great substitute for pasta. Serve with marinara sauce or with olive oil and some of your favorite spices!

Nutrition Facts: Serving size, 1 cup—calories 31, fiber 5 g, protein 1 g, fat 1 g, saturated fat 0 g, carbohydrate 7 g, cholesterol 0 mg, sodium 17 mg, sugars 11 g.

WILTED CABBAGE

serves six (2g fiber/serving)

- 1 teaspoon olive oil
- 6 cups savoy cabbage or Chinese cabbage
- ¼ cup low-sodium chicken stock
- Fresh ground black pepper
- ½ teaspoon cumin seeds
- 2 teaspoons apple cider vinegar

Heat oil in a Dutch oven over medium heat. Add cabbage and stock and cook about 3–4 minutes until cabbage starts to wilt, stirring occasionally. Stir in pepper. Put cumin seeds in a small saucepan and toast over medium heat 1 minute, shaking pan frequently. Add seeds and apple cider vinegar to cabbage and cook 3 more minutes until tender, stirring occasionally.

Brenda's Tips: There are many varieties of cabbage, and you can use any of your favorites for this dish.

Nutrition Facts: Serving size, 1 cup—calories 27, fiber 2 g, protein 1 g, fat 1 g, saturated fat 0 g, carbohydrate 5 g, cholesterol 0 mg, sodium 20 mg, sugars 2 g.

DESSERT RECIPES

Just in case you have a craving for something sweet, here are some dessert recipes that are healthy, are low-calorie, and have a good amount of fiber.

DARK SWEET CHERRIES WITH WHIPPED CREAM

serves one (3g fiber/serving)

- 1 cup dark sweet cherries (frozen)
- 1 tablespoon whipped cream

Measure out 1 cup of cherries. Let thaw (or microwave 30 seconds). Top with whipped cream.

Brenda's Tips: The dark sweet cherries are sweeter than lighter sweet cherries, but whichever kind you prefer is fine.

Nutrition Facts: One serving—calories 118, fiber 3 g, protein 1 g.

APPLE CRISP

serves four (2g fiber/serving)

- 2 cup red apples peeled, cored, and sliced very thin
- 2 tablespoons olive oil
- 2 teaspoons cinnamon
- 1 teaspoon vanilla extract
- ½ teaspoon fresh nutmeg
- ¼ cup fruit/nut granola

Preheat oven to 350°F.

Place a very thin layer of apples; then olive oil; then cinnamon, vanilla, and nutmeg evenly in a shallow glass baking dish. Then do another layer the same way. Top with granola and bake 30–40 minutes, until apples are tender and the edges are bubbly.

Brenda's Tips: This dish is low in calories and has no fat, but it makes you feel as though you've eaten apple cobbler.

Nutrition Facts: One serving (¼ recipe)—calories 127, fiber 2 g, protein 1 g.

CARROT SPICE SNACK CAKE

serves twelve (2g fiber/serving)

- ½ cup liquid honey

- 3 tablespoons cooking oil

- 2 eggs

- 1 cup spelt flour

- ½ teaspoon sea salt

- ¾ teaspoon baking soda

- 1 teaspoon baking powder

- 1 teaspoon cinnamon

- 1 teaspoon fresh grated nutmeg

- 2 cups grated carrots

- ¼ cup applesauce (unsweetened)

- ¼ cup chopped walnuts

- 7 ounces unsweetened
  crushed pineapple

- Cooking spray

Preheat oven to 300°F.

Using a mixer, beat honey, cooking oil, and eggs together until well blended. Add flour, salt, baking soda, baking powder, cinnamon, and nutmeg; mix well. Fold in carrots, applesauce, nuts, and pineapple. Spray an 8- by 8-inch ungreased pan with cooking spray. Add cake mixture to pan. Bake in preheated oven for 50–60 minutes.

Nutrition Facts: One serving (¼ cake)—calories 124, fiber 2 g, protein 3 g.

MANGO SORBET

serves eight (1g fiber/serving)

- ¼ cup SweetLife brand all-natural sweetener

- ¾ cup water

- 2 ripe mangoes (about ½ pound each)

- Juice of 1 lime

Combine SweetLife and water in a small saucepan and place over low heat. Stir until SweetLife dissolves completely and syrup is clear. Remove from heat and allow to cool to room temperature.

Peel mango and cut away from the pit. Combine mango, lime juice, and syrup in blender or food processor. Blend until completely smooth, about 30 seconds. Cover and refrigerate until cold or overnight.

Stir chilled mixture, then freeze in an ice cream freezer. Follow the manufacturer's instructions.

Brenda's Tips: Remember—you can increase the fiber content by adding sprinkle table fiber.

Nutrition Facts: One serving (⅛ recipe)—calories 80, fiber 1 g, protein 0 g.

SNACK IDEAS

Use any of these snack ideas during Phase One and Phase Two of the Fiber35 Diet Plan. They are all from 100 to 150 calories each and contain fiber and protein. Or make up your own ideas—just be sure to include fiber and protein.

Snack Bars

Try to find a bar that has both fiber and protein: preferably 10 grams of fiber, 10 grams of protein, and approximately 200 calories per bar. You can use half of this bar as a 100-calorie snack during Phase One and Phase Two of the diet.

Miscellaneous Snacks

Pineapple and Cottage Cheese

• ½ cup fresh pineapple and 3 ounces low-fat cottage cheese

Note: Remember that any raw fruits or vegetables can be used as a snack in all phases of the Fiber35 Diet plan. Try to choose ones with the highest fiber content. Check the fiber chart in Chapter 5 before shopping.

Nutrition Facts: Calories 100, fiber 1 g, protein 12 g.

Apple with Almond Butter

• ½ medium apple, sliced, with 1 tablespoon almond butter

Nutrition Facts: Calories 145, fiber 3.5 g, protein 2.5 g.

Raspberries and Cottage Cheese

• ½ cup raspberries with 3 ounces low-fat cottage cheese

Nutrition Facts: Calories 100, fiber 4 g, protein 12 g.

Brown Rice Cake with Almond Butter

• 1 brown rice cake with 1 teaspoon almond butter

Nutrition Facts: Calories 144, fiber 4 g, protein 5 g.

Celery and Hummus

- 2 ribs celery with 1 ounce (2 tablespoons) homemade hummus
  (see recipe following)

Nutrition Facts: Calories 85, fiber 3.5 g, protein 4 g.

Crackers and Guacamole

- 2 flax crackers with 2 ounces homemade guacamole
  (see recipe following)

Nutrition Facts: Calories 132, fiber 7.5 g, protein 3 g.

Tortilla Chips and Salsa

- 1 ounce blue corn tortilla chips (15 chips) and 2 ounces (4 tablespoons) homemade salsa
  (see recipe following)

Nutrition Facts: Calories 150, fiber 3 g, protein 3 g.

Crackers and Egg Salad

- 2 flax crackers with 1 ounce (2 tablespoons) homemade egg salad
  (see recipe following)

Nutrition Facts: Calories 100, fiber 4.5 g, protein 5 g.

Popcorn

- 4 cups air-popped corn

Nutrition Facts: Calories 130, fiber 6 g, protein 3 g.

Smoked Tuna and Celery

- 2 tablespoons smoked tuna spread and 2 ribs celery

Nutrition Facts: Calories 100, fiber 2 g, protein 3.5 g.

Celery and Tuna Salad

- 2 ribs celery with 1 ounce (2 tablespoons) homemade tuna salad
  (see recipe following)

Nutrition Facts: Calories 60, fiber 2 g, protein 7 g.

TURKEY SANDWICH

serves two   (2g fiber/serving)

- 2 slices whole grain bread

- 1 slice deli turkey

- 1 teaspoon mustard

- 1 large leaf lettuce

- 2 slices tomato

Nutrition Facts: Serving size, ½ sandwich—calories 103, fiber 2 g, protein 5 g, fat 2 g, saturated fat 0 g, carbohydrate 16 g, cholesterol 5 mg, sodium 292 mg, sugars 5 g.

ROASTED RED PEPPER HUMMUS DIP

(1.5g fiber/serving)

- One 7-ounce jar roasted red peppers

- One 15-ounce can chickpeas, rinsed and drained

- One 15-ounce can cannellini (white kidney) beans, drained and rinsed

- ¼ cup tahini

- 3 garlic cloves, minced

- 2 tablespoons fresh lemon juice

- 1 teaspoon ground cumin

- 2 tablespoons low-fat plain yogurt

- Sea salt and pepper to taste

Mix all ingredients except salt and pepper in a food processor. Process until mixture is smooth.

Season with salt and pepper.

Cover and refrigerate. Serve chilled or at room temperature.

Brenda's Tip: This is better the next day!

Nutrition Facts: Serving size, 1 ounce—calories 65, fiber 1.5 g, protein 3 g, fat 2 g, saturated fat 0 g, carbohydrate 9 g, cholesterol 0 mg, sodium 110 mg, sugars 2 g.

HOMEMADE SALSA

(1g fiber/serving)

- 2 large tomatoes, seeded and chopped
- 1 serrano or jalepeño pepper, chopped
- ⅓ cup chopped green onion
- 2 tablespoons chopped fresh cilantro
- 2 tablespoons fresh lime juice
- ¼ teaspoon salt

Mix all ingredients well and chill.

Nutrition Facts: Serving size, 2 ounces—calories 13, fiber 1 g, protein 1 g, fat 0 g, saturated fat 0 g, carbohydrate 4 g, cholesterol 0 mg, sodium 100 mg, sugars 2 g.

HOMEMADE GUACAMOLE

(3g fiber/serving)

- 3 large Haas avocados, ripe
- ½ red onion, chopped
- 2 cloves garlic, minced
- 1 teaspoon ground cumin
- 2 small limes, juiced
- 2 tablespoons chopped cilantro
- 4 green onions, sliced thin

Cut avocados in half and remove pulp; mash well in bowl. Add all other ingredients and mix well. Chill.

Nutrition Facts: Serving size, 2 ounces—calories 72, fiber 3 g, protein 1 g, fat 6 g, saturated fat 0 g, carbohydrate 5 g, cholesterol 0 mg, sodium 5 mg, sugars 1 g.

EGG SALAD

(0g fiber/serving)

- 1 boiled egg, whole
- 1 boiled egg, white only
- ½ teaspoon dry mustard
- ½ tablespoon light mayonnaise
- ½ tablespoon pickle relish
- Pepper to taste

Place eggs in small bowl and mash with fork. Add remaining ingredients and mix well. Chill.

Nutrition Facts: Serving size, 1 ounce—calories 46, fiber 0 g, protein 3 g, fat 3 g, saturated fat 1 g, carbohydrate 2 g, cholesterol 70 mg, sodium 80 mg, sugars 1 g.

HEALTHY TUNA SALAD

(0g fiber/serving)

- 1 small can light tuna in water, drained
- 1 tablespoon light mayonnaise
- ½ tablespoon pickle relish
- 2 slices of fresh apple, chopped
- ½ teaspoon celery seed
- Black pepper to taste

Mix all ingredients well and chill.

Nutrition Facts: Serving size, 1 ounce—calories 40, fiber 0 g, protein 6 g, fat 1 g, saturated fat 0 g, carbohydrate 1 g, cholesterol 8 mg, sodium 35 mg, sugars 0 g

DRINK IDEAS TO GET THE WATER YOU NEED DAILY

Alternatives to water include herbal teas. Celestial Seasonings Red Zinger and the berry teas are really good choices. You can make these in large containers to store in your refrigerator, ready to drink as you would iced tea.

You can also add fresh lemon or lime juice to make water a little more enjoyable, and for a change from plain water.

Do not count caffeinated drinks like soda or coffee as part of your water intake.

It is important not to drink water directly from the tap, as most city water has many added components, like fluoride and chlorine, that are not OK. Reverse osmosis is a type of water filter that is fairly inexpensive and easy to install on your kitchen sink. These systems are available in most areas of the United States. The Brita filters are OK, but reverse osmosis is fairly economical and doesn't require frequent filter changes.

CHAPTER 15

BRINGING YOUR RESOURCES TOGETHER

In this chapter, you'll find shopping tips to help you recognize and mobilize the resources needed to carry out the Fiber35 Diet in a simple and efficient manner. The resources themselves will be found in the Resource Directory. I've also provided samples of weekly menus for each phase of the diet. These should help you craft your own daily menus and make sense out of all your options.

THE SHOPPING LIST

Regardless of where you shop and whether you shop just once a week or daily, you'll always want to prepare a shopping list. Shopping with a list will make your trip more efficient and will help you to do less impulse buying. In the long run, that means fewer unhealthy temptations around the house. It also means that you have prepared beforehand, and preparation takes a lot of the guesswork out of trying to determine the caloric content of foods.

To assist you in your grocery shopping, I've compiled a list of items you'll probably be buying to complete the first two phases, and to continue onward into Phase Three for life. The following list is a guide to common foods recommended in the Fiber35 Diet and in the recipes found in this book. It's a great tool to use as you begin the Fiber35 Diet. You don't necessarily have to go out and buy all the ingredients listed below at the start of your journey. Use your meal plans to help map out which items you'll need in the first week or two, keeping in mind that fresh ingredients won't last more than three to five days. I recommend that you compose your own personal grocery list prior to each trip to the market using the comprehensive one here as your initial guide.

Grains

Amount generally used in the Fiber35 Diet recipes is a ½ cup. These are found in most health food stores.

Brown rice	Millet	Steel-cut oats

Breads

Used in 1- to 2-ounce servings or by the slice. These are found in most health food stores.

Flax crackers	Multigrain breads

Oils

Amount generally used is 1 to 2 tablespoons.

Cooking spray	Peanut oil
Olive oil	Sesame seed oil

Nuts and Seeds

Amount used in the Fiber35 Diet recipes is generally 1 to 2 tablespoons.

Pecans	Raw almonds	Sesame seeds
Pistachios	Raw walnuts	

Spices

Amount used in the Fiber35 Diet recipes is generally ½ to 1 teaspoon.

Bay leaf	Fresh black pepper	Sea salt
Celery seed	Fresh ginger	Thyme
Chili powder	Fresh nutmeg	Turmeric
Cinnamon	Marjoram	Vanilla extract
Cumin	Oregano	
Dried chives	Red pepper flakes	

Dairy Products

Eggs (preferably organic and natural)

Low-fat plain yogurt

Mozzarella cheese

Parmesan cheese

Small container low-fat cottage cheese

Small container ricotta cheese

Fruits

How much fruit you buy will depend on how many shakes a day you are drinking or how many fruit servings you have for snacks. The amounts here are possibilities.

1 avocado

1 lime

1 mango

1 pear

1 small package frozen dark sweet cherries

1 whole pineapple (some to eat fresh and some to freeze)

½ pint blueberries

½ pint raspberries

2 lemons

3 oranges

4 red apples

6 bananas (some to eat fresh and some to freeze)

Several Granny Smith apples

Small container of strawberries

Vegetables

1 bunch asparagus
1 bunch celery
1 bunch cilantro
1 bunch collard greens
1 bunch endive
1 bunch fennel
1 bunch green onions
1 bunch kale
1 bunch or bag of carrots
1 bunch parsley
1 each green, yellow, red pepper
1 ear fresh corn
1 head cauliflower

1 medium butternut squash
1 red onion
1 serrano or jalapeño pepper
1 small container mint leaves
1 small container rosemary leaves
1 Spanish onion
1 sweet onion
1 sweet potato
1 whole bunch bulb garlic
12 snow peas

2 onions
2 radishes
2 tomatoes
3 cups mixed baby greens
4 cups spinach
Small bunch broccoli
Small carton cremini mushrooms
Small container basil leaves
Small container bean sprouts

Meats

½ pound beef, sliced thin
½ pound sliced turkey breast

12 ounces shrimp
2 chicken breasts (boneless, skinless)

2 pounds boneless turkey breast
6 ounces lump crabmeat

Miscellaneous Pantry Items

1 bag blue corn chips

1 container almond milk (found in most health food stores)

1 package rice lasagna noodles

Almond flour

Applesauce (unsweetened)

Baking powder

Balsamic vinegar

Buckwheat flour

Dijon mustard

Dried cherries

Ground flax meal

Honey

Hot sauce

Instant decaf coffee

Light mayonnaise

Light whipping cream

Low-sodium soy sauce

Maple sugar

Pickle relish

Prepared mustard

Red chili

Red lentils

Rice flour

Small bottle maple syrup

Small container almond butter

Small container fresh orange juice

Spelt flour

SweetLife, or other sugar substitute

White wine vinegar

Canned Items

Use low-sodium or no-salt versions of all items listed below.

Black beans

Canned salmon

Cannellini beans

Chicken stock

Diced tomatoes

Green chilis

Red kidney beans

Small can tuna (light, water-packed)

Tomato juice

Unsweetened crushed pineapple

White beans

White kidney beans

Supplements

These items are found in most health food stores.

Colon Cleanse formula to relieve constipation

Fiber wafers to eat before meals

Natural food bars—Fiber/protein bars (try to find bars that have at least 10 grams of fiber and 10 grams of protein)

Protein and fiber shakes (try to find shakes that have 20 grams of protein and 10 grams of fiber)

Sprinkle fiber—a natural soluble fiber that dissolves clearly in drinks, soups, and sauces

PICKING YOUR MARKET

People generally tend to spend more time—and money—picking out shoes or clothing than they do selecting their food.

Cleanliness is of utmost importance in choosing a store. Stores should look clean and smell appealing. A spotless store means little risk of health problems and, in general, reflects the managers' attitude toward their merchandise, as well as toward their customers.

Get to know shopkeepers and department managers. Don't be afraid to ask them to get something they do not already have. Most shops will be willing to special-order items for you. The grocery business is very competitive. Stores want your business. Remember—you can shop anywhere. Use this fact to your advantage to provide something approaching one-stop shopping for your convenience.

Also, for specialty foods, pick the best shop for your needs. You may choose to limit your bakery purchases to a bakery that makes specialty artisan loaves or breads that meet your dietary criteria. Find a place where you can buy the best-quality meats and the freshest fish. This may mean an extra stop outside your regular grocery, but the quality of your purchases will make it more than worthwhile.

Read labels! If you can't pronounce an ingredient, don't buy the product! Chemical additives stress the liver, impairing your fat-burning potential.

Your Shopping Options

Today we have an unprecedented number of healthy shopping options, such as organic food co-ops and mega health food markets. Here's the lowdown on some of these options.

Natural Foods Stores and Supermarkets

There are currently many national and regional chains of natural food supermarkets. Many of these are hybrid stores that combine natural, conventional, and gourmet foods. Look for stores that have a wide range of merchandise; salad and juice bars; meat, poultry, and fish; and a section of prepared foods with healthy choices in case you want to pick up one or several meals without having to cook. Many of these stores have extensive dietary supplement sections. These are the type of stores that can easily become one-stop shops, or at least the shop from which you will get the majority of your food.

Health Food Stores

These are usually owner-operated stores that are smaller than natural food supermarkets. Because they are owner-operated, they can cater to your individual needs if this is where you choose to shop. These stores carry nutritional supplements and are usually a good source of bulk foods. Most carry organic produce.

Supermarkets

Many conventional grocery stores now carry organic produce and natural products in addition to the foods they have traditionally sold. Some of them have whole sections called "stores within a store" where they modify the building with a wood floor and trim so that it has the appearance and merchandise of a high-end natural foods store.

If you want your grocer to carry more natural products, or if there are specific things that you want, remember to let the management know!

Farmers' Markets and Fruit Stands

These are great sources for the freshest seasonal produce and products. Many have organic selections. You can also find regional specialty items like honey, jellies, jams, and some prepared desserts, breads, and dairy products. Many of these businesses also sell fresh herbs and spices.

Organic Produce Home Delivery

This is an up-and-coming service for busy people. Most delivery services provide whatever produce is ripe and available. The extra time you gain by not having to go out to shop can be spent thinking of creative ways to use what the service sells, which will vary with the seasons. See Resource Directory for some ideas.

Co-ops

Some people organize into groups that contract to buy products from local organic growers and food distributors. They use the buying power of a group to get products at wholesale prices. Through a well-organized co-op, you can obtain organic meats, poultry, and dairy items that are not found in most stores. Organic produce can often be obtained through this method at the same price as conventional produce from a regular grocery store, or at a lower price. This is a great way to support small local business and build community. Like home delivery services, co-ops get the freshest possible foods but don't have much control over the produce selection from week to week.

Bakeries

You can find bakeries that make whatever your heart desires: whole grain breads, non-gluten breads, and breads made from traditional grains such as millet, quinoa, or spelt. If ordered in bulk, these breads can be purchased at a discount and then frozen for later use. See Resource Directory.

Fish Markets

The fresher the better when it comes to fish. Choose the cleanest fish market available (your nose is usually a good indicator of freshness). If you don't live near water, find out where you can buy the freshest fish locally. Find out when fresh shipments come in, and plan your fish meals around those days.

Butchers

Find butchers who are progressively phasing in the cleaner, healthier meats (steroid-free and antibiotic-free beef and poultry products) that are becoming more readily available. I strongly recommend patronizing markets that carry such items. Learn the differences between free-range, cage-free, and grass-fed. You will be amazed at how different some of these meats will taste from the meat of animals that were conventionally raised and fed.

Mail Order

You can now purchase a wide variety of high-quality foods and food products through the mail or online, including specialty meats, fruit, and other specialty items.

Summary

I suggest that you make a plan before shopping, including preparing and using a grocery list. Choose your stores well, and use management to help you get the food items you want. Be aware of and use the other options that are available to you, such as co-ops, bakeries, fruit and vegetable stands, and mail order. Choose meat and poultry suppliers who offer progressive options like hormone-free and antibiotic-free meats. Buy the freshest fish available.

THE Fiber 35 Diet

SAMPLE WEEKLY MENUS

The following pages contain sample menus for each phase of the Fiber35 Diet. Don't be afraid to use these as a guide only and mix and match your meals however you like, so long as you stay within your caloric boundaries and get at least 35 grams of fiber a day. Enjoy!

PHASE 1 THE FIBER35 DIET – SUGGESTED WEEKLY MEAL PLAN

	Monday	Tuesday	Wednesday
Breakfast	**Chocolate Mocha Madness Shake** **Coffee or tea**	**Steel-Cut Oat Crunch** **Coffee or tea**	**Spinach & Chèvre Omelet or Protein-fiber shake** **Coffee or tea**
	Fiber: 10 g Calories: 225	*Fiber: 12 g Calories: 312*	*Fiber: 3 g Calories: 220*
Snack	**1 protein-fiber bar**	**Dark Sweet Cherries with Whipped Cream**	**1 protein-fiber bar**
	Fiber: 10 g Calories: 200	*Fiber: 3 g Calories: 118*	*Fiber: 10 g Calories: 200*
Lunch	**Seafood, Spinach, and Orange Salad** **Herbal tea**	**Orange Pineapple Crave Shake** **2 flax crackers with Egg Salad**	**Big Salad and ½ Turkey Sandwich** **Herbal tea**
	Fiber: 6 g Calories: 245	*Fiber: 14.5 g Calories: 380*	*Fiber: 12 g Calories: 403*
Snack	**½ protein-fiber bar**	**½ protein-fiber bar**	**½ protein-fiber bar**
	Fiber: 5 g Calories: 100	*Fiber: 5 g Calories: 100*	*Fiber: 5 g Calories: 100*
Dinner	**West Indies Wild Salmon with Brown Rice** **Herbal tea**	**Seared Chicken with Greens, Raspberries, and Pear** **Herbal tea**	**1 cup Vegetable Bean Chili with ½ cup brown rice** **Herbal tea**
	Fiber: 5 g Calories: 469	*Fiber: 6 g Calories: 299*	*Fiber: 16 g Calories: 366*
Snack	**½ cup Raspberries Low Fat Cottage Cheese**	**½ protein-fiber bar**	**½ cup Raspberries with Low Fat Cottage Cheese**
	Fiber: 4 g Calories: 100	*Fiber: 5 g Calories: 100*	*Fiber: 4 g Calories: 100*
Daily Totals	*Fiber: 40 g* *Calories: 1338*	*Fiber: 45.5 g* *Calories: 1309*	*Fiber: 50 g* *Calories: 1389*
Fiber Flush Bonus	*Daily calories 1338* *Fiber 40 x 7 = 280* *Net calories 1058*	*Daily calories 1309* *Fiber 45.5 x 7 = 318* *Net calories 991*	*Daily calories 1389* *Fiber 50 x 7 = 350* *Net calories 1039*

Metabolic Boosters 5-7 daily: Choose from frequent eating, muscle boosting, aerobic exercise, water, eight hours of sleep, sauna, and detoxification.

Thursday	Friday	Saturday	Sunday
Orange Pineapple Crave Shake **Coffee or tea**	**1 cup Millet Porridge** **Coffee or tea**	**Raspberry Delight Shake** **Coffee or tea**	**Multigrain French Toast with Yogurt and Bananas** **Coffee or tea**
Fiber: 10 g Calories: 280	*Fiber: 7 g Calories: 262*	*Fiber: 14 g Calories: 220*	*Fiber: 6 g Calories: 295*
1 protein-fiber bar	**½ protein-fiber bar**	**2 flax crackers with Guacamole**	**½ protein-fiber bar**
Fiber: 10 g Calories: 200	*Fiber: 5 g Calories: 100*	*Fiber: 7.5 g Calories: 132*	*Fiber: 5 g Calories: 100*
Mixed Salad with Chicken, Fruit, and Nuts (½ serving) **Herbal tea**	**Butternut Squash Soup** **½ Turkey Sandwich** **Herbal tea**	**Chicken Wraps** **Herbal tea**	**Chocolate Banana Dream Shake** **2 tablespoons Smoked Tuna Spread with Celery** **Herbal tea**
Fiber: 2.5 g Calories: 229	*Fiber: 7 g Calories: 262*	*Fiber: 2 g Calories: 305*	*Fiber:14 g Calories: 350*
1 protein-fiber bar	**Dark Sweet Cherries with Whipped Cream**	**½ protein-fiber bar**	**2 Ribs Celery with 1 ounce Roasted Red Pepper Hummus Dip**
Fiber: 10g Calories: 200	*Fiber: 3 g Calories: 118*	*Fiber: 5g Calories: 100*	*Fiber: 3.5 Calories: 85*
Grilled Chicken Kabobs **1 cup Spaghetti Squash** **Herbal tea**	**½ Greens and Beans Salad** **Turkey Burger** **Herbal tea**	**Turkey Roll Stuffed with Goat Cheese and Spinach** **Steamed veggie** **Herbal tea**	**Asian Chicken with Bok Choy and ½ cup brown rice** **Herbal tea**
Fiber: 6 g Calories: 178	*Fiber: 13 g Calories: 443*	*Fiber: 7 g Calories: 430*	*Fiber: 4 g Calories: 307*
Dark Sweet Cherries with Whipped Cream	**½ cup Pineapple with 3 ounces Low-Fat Cottage Cheese**	**½ protein-fiber bar**	**1 Medium Apple with 1 tablespoon Almond Butter**
Fiber: 3 g Calories: 118	*Fiber: 1 g Calories: 100*	*Fiber: 5 g Calories: 100*	*Fiber: 2.5 g Calories: 141*
Fiber: 41.5 g *Calories: 1205*	*Fiber: 36 g* *Calories: 1285*	*Fiber: 40.5 g* *Calories: 1287*	*Fiber: 35 g* *Calories: 1278*
Daily calories 1205 *Fiber 41.5 x 7 = 290* *Net calories 915*	*Daily calories 1285* *Fiber 36 x 7 = 252* *Net calories 1033*	*Daily calories 1287* *Fiber 40.5 x 7 = 283* *Net calories 1004*	*Daily calories 1278* *Fiber 35 x 7 = 245* *Net calories 1033*

PHASE 2 THE FIBER35 DIET– SUGGESTED WEEKLY MEAL PLAN

		Monday	Tuesday	Wednesday
Breakfast		Chocolate Peanut Butter Banana Blitz Shake Coffee or tea	Blueberry Almond and Flax Buckwheat Pancakes Coffee or tea	Fresh Fruit Parfait Coffee or tea
		Fiber: 12 g Calories: 285	*Fiber: 7 g Calories: 326*	*Fiber: 10 g Calories: 351*
Snack		1 protein-fiber bar	1 ounce Blue Corn Tortilla Chips with 2 ounces Salsa	Chocolate Banana Dream Shake
		Fiber: 10 g Calories: 200	*Fiber: 4 g Calories: 163*	*Fiber: 12 g Calories: 250*
Lunch		Layered Black Bean Salad and ½ Turkey Sandwich Herbal tea	Big Salad Tomato Basil Soup Herbal tea	Vegetable Bean Chili Big Salad Herbal tea
		Fiber: 19 g Calories: 427	*Fiber: 12 g Calories: 349*	*Fiber: 24 g Calories: 558*
Snack		1 protein-fiber bar	Chocolate Mocha Madness Shake	½ protein-fiber bar
		Fiber: 10 g Calories: 200	*Fiber: 10 g Calories: 225*	*Fiber: 5 g Calories: 100*
Dinner		Beef and Vegetable Fried Rice Herbal tea	Vegetable Lasagna Herbal tea	Zesty Lemon Herb Turkey Breast, Southern Kale, Cauliflower Mash Herbal tea
		Fiber: 4 g Calories: 437	*Fiber: 4 g Calories: 483*	*Fiber: 4 g Calories: 342*
Snack		Apple Crisp	1 protein-fiber bar	Dark Sweet Cherries with Whipped Cream
		Fiber: 2 g Calories: 127	*Fiber: 10 g Calories: 200*	*Fiber: 3 g Calories: 118*
Daily Totals		*Fiber: 57 g* *Calories: 1676*	*Fiber: 47 g* *Calories: 1745*	*Fiber: 58 g* *Calories: 1719*
Fiber Flush Bonus		*Daily calories 1676* *Fiber 57 × 7 = 399* *Net calories 1227*	*Daily calories 1745* *Fiber 47 × 7 = 329* *Net calories 1416*	*Daily calories 1719* *Fiber 58 × 7 = 406* *Net calories 1313*

Metabolic Boosters 4–6 daily: Choose from frequent eating, muscle boosting, aerobic exercise, water, eight hours of sleep, sauna, and detoxification.

Thursday	Friday	Saturday	Sunday
Salmon Frittata **Coffee or tea**	**Steel-Cut Oat Crunch** **Coffee or tea**	**Millet Porridge** **Coffee or tea**	**Multigrain French Toast with Yogurt and Bananas** **Coffee or tea**
Fiber: 5 g Calories: 260	*Fiber: 12 g Calories: 312*	*Fiber: 7 g Calories: 262*	*Fiber: 6 g Calories: 295*
Orange Pineapple Crave Shake	**1 protein-fiber shake or bar**	**1 protein-fiber shake or bar**	**1 protein-fiber shake or bar**
Fiber: 10 g Calories: 280	*Fiber: 10 g Calories: 200*	*Fiber: 10 g Calories: 200*	*Fiber: 10 g Calories: 200*
Crab and White Bean Salad **Turkey Sandwich** **Butternut Squash Soup** **Herbal tea**	**Greens and Beans Salad** **3 ounces Chicken Breast** **Herbal tea**	**Mixed Salad with Chicken, Fruit, and Nuts** **Herbal tea**	**Seafood Spinach and Orange Salad with Whole Grain Bread** **Herbal tea**
Fiber: 13 g Calories: 487	*Fiber: 12 g Calories: 404*	*Fiber: 5 g Calories: 458*	*Fiber: 11 g Calories: 337*
1 medium apple with **1 tablespoon almond butter**	**2 flax crackers with Homemade Guacamole**	**½ cup Pineapple with 3 ounces Low-Fat Cottage Cheese**	**2 ounces Healthy Tuna Salad** **1 ounce flax crackers**
Fiber: 2.5 g Calories: 141	*Fiber: 7.5 g Calories: 132*	*Fiber: 1 g Calories: 100*	*Fiber: 8 g Calories: 146*
Red Lentil Soup with **½ Turkey Sandwich** **Herbal tea**	**Pistachio-Crusted Chicken and Smashed Sweet Potatoes** **Herbal tea**	**Seared Chicken with Greens, Raspberries and Pear with ½ cup brown rice** **Herbal tea**	**Black Bean Soup** **Spinach Salad** **Herbal tea**
Fiber: 13 g Calories: 491	*Fiber: 8 g Calories: 456*	*Fiber: 8 g Calories: 407*	*Fiber: 24 g Calories: 445*
Apple Crisp	**protein-fiber bar or shake**	**Carrot Spice Snack Cake (2 servings)**	**½ cup Pineapple with 3 ounces Low-Fat Cottage Cheese**
Fiber: 2 g Calories: 127	*Fiber: 10 g Calories: 200*	*Fiber: 4 g Calories: 248*	*Fiber: 1 g Calories: 100*
Fiber: 45.5 g *Calories: 1786*	*Fiber: 59.5 g* *Calories: 1704*	*Fiber: 35 g* *Calories: 1675*	*Fiber: 60 g* *Calories: 1523*
Daily calories 1786 *Fiber 45.5 × 7 = 318* *Net calories 1468*	*Daily calories 1704* *Fiber 59.5 × 7 = 416* *Net calories 1288*	*Daily calories 1675* *Fiber 35 × 7 = 245* *Net calories 1430*	*Daily calories 1523* *Fiber 60 × 7 = 420* *Net calories 1103*

PHASE 3 THE FIBER35 DIET – SUGGESTED WEEKLY MEAL PLAN

		Monday	Tuesday	Wednesday
Breakfast		Blueberry Almond and Flax Buckwheat Pancakes (5 Pancakes) Coffee or tea	Steel-Cut Oat Crunch with Boiled Egg Coffee or tea	Orange Pineapple Crave Shake and protein-fiber bar Coffee or tea
		Fiber: 11.5 g Calories: 540	*Fiber: 12 g Calories: 392*	*Fiber: 20 g Calories: 480*
Snack		Celery (4 Stalks) Hummus Dip (4 tablespoons)	Chocolate Banana Dream Shake	1 medium apple with 1 tablespoon almond butter
		Fiber: 7 g Calories: 170	*Fiber: 12 g Calories: 250*	*Fiber: 2.5 g Calories: 141*
Lunch		Turkey Sandwich Herbal tea	Big Salad with Grilled Chicken Breast Herbal tea	Grilled Chicken Kabobs Southern Kale 1 cup brown rice Herbal tea
		Fiber: 4 g Calories: 206	*Fiber: 10 g Calories: 531*	*Fiber: 9 g Calories: 479*
Snack		1 protein-fiber bar	2 flax crackers with Homemade Egg Salad	1 protein-fiber bar
		Fiber: 10 g Calories: 200	*Fiber: 4.5 g Calories: 100*	*Fiber: 10 g Calories: 200*
Dinner		Chicken Marsala 1 cup brown rice Roasted Broccoli with Lemon and Shallots Herbal tea	Pistachio-Crusted Chicken with Smashed Sweet Potatoes Herbal tea	Beef and Vegetable Fried Rice Herbal tea
		Fiber: 8 g Calories: 582	*Fiber: 8 g Calories: 456*	*Fiber: 4 g Calories: 437*
Snack		½ cup Raspberries with Low-Fat Cottage Cheese	Mango Sorbet	Dove's Dark Chocolate Squares (2)
		Fiber: 4 g Calories: 100	*Fiber: 1 g Calories: 80*	*Fiber: 0 g Calories: 84*
Daily Totals		*Fiber: 44.5 g* *Calories: 1618*	*Fiber: 47.5 g* *Calories: 1809*	*Fiber: 45.5 g* *Calories: 1821*
Fiber Flush Bonus		*Daily calories 1618* *Fiber 44.5 × 7 = 311* *Net calories 1307*	*Daily calories 1809* *Fiber 47.5 × 7 = 332* *Net calories 1477*	*Daily calories 1821* *Fiber 45.5 × 7 = 318* *Net calories 1503*

Metabolic Boosters 3-4 daily: Choose from frequent eating, muscle boosting, aerobic exercise, water, eight hours of sleep, sauna, and detoxification.

Thursday	Friday	Saturday	Sunday
Salmon Frittata **1 slice multigrain toast** **1 pat butter** **Coffee or tea**	**Fresh Fruit Parfait** **Coffee or tea**	**Millet Porridge** **1 Boiled Egg** **Coffee or tea**	**Multigrain French Toast with Yogurt and Bananas** **Coffee or tea**
Fiber: 7 g Calories: 376	*Fiber: 10 g Calories: 351*	*Fiber: 7 g Calories: 339*	*Fiber: 6 g Calories: 295*
Chocolate Peanut Butter Banana Blitz Shake	**½ cup Pineapple with 3 ounces Low-Fat Cottage Cheese**	**4 tablespoons Smoked Tuna Spread with 4 Stalks Celery**	**4 cups air-popped Popcorn** **2 pats butter**
Fiber: 12 g Calories: 285	*Fiber: 1 g Calories: 100*	*Fiber: 4 g Calories: 200*	*Fiber: 6 g Calories: 202*
Zesty Chicken Patties **Big Salad** **Herbal tea**	**White Bean Stew** **Big Salad** **Herbal tea**	**Chicken Asparagus Stir Fry with 1 cup cooked brown rice** **Herbal tea**	**2 cups Vegetable Soup** **Turkey Sandwich** **Herbal tea**
Fiber: 11 g Calories: 572	*Fiber: 25 g Calories: 624*	*Fiber: 9 g Calories: 541*	*Fiber: 12 g Calories: 390*
protein-fiber bar or shake	**protein-fiber bar or shake**	**Orange Pineapple Crave Shake**	**Chocolate Banana Dream Shake**
Fiber: 10 g Calories: 200	*Fiber: 10 g Calories: 200*	*Fiber: 10 g Calories: 280*	*Fiber: 12 g Calories: 250*
Chicken Marsala **Spaghetti Squash** **Herbal tea**	**Chicken Cacciatore** **Wilted Cabbage** **1 cup brown rice** **Herbal tea**	**Baked Fish** **1 medium baked sweet potato with 2 pats butter** **Herbal tea**	**Wild Salmon with Citrus Marinade** **Medley of Roasted Vegetables** **Cauliflower Mash** **Herbal tea**
Fiber: 6 g Calories: 300	*Fiber: 11 g Calories: 442*	*Fiber: 8 g Calories: 343*	*Fiber: 6 g Calories: 423*
Carrot Spice Cake (1 serving)	**Apple Crisp (1 serving)**	**protein-fiber bar or shake**	**protein-fiber bar or shake**
Fiber: 2 g Calories: 124	*Fiber: 2 g Calories: 127*	*Fiber: 10 g Calories: 200*	*Fiber: 10 g Calories: 200*
Fiber: 48 g *Calories: 1857*	*Fiber: 59 g* *Calories: 1844*	*Fiber: 48 g* *Calories: 1903*	*Fiber: 52 g* *Calories: 1760*
Daily calories 1857 *Fiber 48 × 7 = 336* *Net calories 1521*	*Daily calories 1844* *Fiber 59 × 7 = 413* *Net calories 1431*	*Daily calories 1903* *Fiber 48 × 7 = 336* *Net calories 1567*	*Daily calories 1760* *Fiber 52 × 7 = 364* *Net calories 1396*

ACKNOWLEDGMENTS

This book is a result of the extraordinary efforts of many wonderful people, without whom The Fiber35 Diet could not have been written. I want to extend my personal and heartfelt thanks to: Bonnie Solow, my literary agent, for her exceptional talent and meticulous attention to detail—her unwavering support has allowed me to share my personal message of nutrition with people worldwide; all of my many friends and colleagues at Free Press, including Martha K. Levin, Dominick V. Anfuso, Suzanne Donahue, Carisa Hays, Sue Fleming, Eric Fuentecilla, Erich Hobbing, Laura Ferguson, Alexandra Noya, and Maria Bruk Aupérin, as well as their outstanding sales force; Dr. Leonard Smith, a wonderful surgeon with a superior intellect and an unmatched compassion for people; Steven Beckman, a special partner and friend, for his passion in bringing this book to fruition; my son, Travis, for all of his hard work and contributions to this book; my daughter, Joy, for her support and patience; Suzin Stockton, for her work on all of my books and projects; Brenda Valen, my assistant, for her teamwork and dedication; Sandee Kiser, my sister, for all her creativity on the recipes; Katie Hagen, for all her work in developing the exercise routines; Tony Tiano, Lennlee Keep, Eli Brown, and the entire team at Santa Fe Productions; WEDU and the Public Broadcasting Service (PBS-TV); Michael Black, Jason Oakman, and the team at Black Sun Studio; and Bonnie Cooper, Jerry Adams, Paul Pavlovich, Pamela Sapio, and Kristin Loberg, for playing a part in all the elements that come together in a book.

Most of all, to my husband, Stan, without whose constant support and love this book would not be complete—thank you for believing so passionately in me.

APPENDIX A

Personal Mission Statement

_____

_____

_____

_____

_____

_____

_____

_____

_____

_____

_____

_____

_____

_____

_____

_____

_____

_____

_____

_____

_____

_____

_____

_____

_____

_____

_____

_____

_____

_____

APPENDIX B

The Fiber35 Diet Daily Journal: **Date:** _____

Meals	Calories	Fiber (grams)
Breakfast		
Snack		
Lunch		
Snack		
Dinner		
Snack		
Supplements		

Daily Total:

Fiber Flush Effect:
multiply: (daily total grams fiber × 7)

Net Calories:
subtract: (daily total calories – fiber flush effect)

APPENDIX C

Resource Directory

Note: The following list of resources is intended as a guide to get you started. It is by no means exhaustive because it's impossible to list every trusted resource available to you. Explore options in your local area, and I invite you to also go to www.fiber35diet.com for updated information and help in finding the best supplements and products to support your health.

Bakeries

DeLand Bakery (whole grain and vegetable breads)
933 North Woodland Boulevard
DeLand, FL 32720
386-734-7553
www.delandbakery.com

Foods Alive (flax crackers)
4840 County Road #4
Waterloo, IN 46793-9770
260-488-4497
www.foodsalive.com

Sami's Pita Bakery (flax crackers)
4920 East Busch Boulevard
Tampa, FL 33617
813-989-2722 or 1-877-989-2722
www.samisbakery.com

Beans and Legumes (Organic)

Eden Foods
701 Tecumseh Road
Clinton, MI 49236
1-888-424-3336
www.edenfoods.com

Westbrae Natural
Westbrae Consumer Relations
The Hain Celestial Group
4600 Sleepytime Drive
Boulder, CO 80301
1-800-434-4246
www.westbrae.com

Broths (Chicken, Vegetable—Low Sodium)

Pacific Natural Foods
19480 Southwest 97th Avenue
Tualatin, OR 97062
503-692-9666 Consumer Affairs ext. 1124
www.pacificfoods.com

Cereals and Grains (whole grain, organic, and gluten-free)

Arrowhead Mills
Arrowhead Mills Consumer Relations
The Hain Celestial Group
4600 Sleepytime Drive
Boulder, CO 80301
1-800-434-4246
www.arrowheadmills.com

Health Valley
www.healthvalley.com

Kashi Company
P.O. Box 8557
La Jolla, CA 92038
858-274-8870
www.kashi.com

Lundberg Family Farms
5370 Church Street
Richvale, CA 95974
530-882-4551
www.lundberg.com

Colon Hydrotherapy

International Association for Colon Hydrotherapy (I-ACT)
P.O. Box 461285
San Antonio, TX 78246-1285
210-366-2888
www.i-act.org

Environmental Products

HealthyHome.com
2894 22nd Avenue North
St. Petersburg, FL 33713
727-322-1058
www.healthyhome.com

Exercise Resistance Bands

Simple Fitness Solutions
1-866-283-4242
www.simplefitnesssolutions.com

Exercise Bands
1-800-500-1979
www.exercisebands.com

Fish (Wild, Fresh, Frozen, and Canned)

Vital Choice Seafood
605 30th Street
Anacortes, WA 98221
1-800-608-4825
www.vitalchoice.com

Fruit (Fresh, Organic—Year-Round)

Cushman Fruit Company
3325 Forest Hill Boulevard
West Palm Beach, FL 33406
1-800-776-7575
www.honeybell.com

Mack's Groves
1-800-327-3525 or 954-941-4528
www.macksgrove.com

Government Agencies

Centers for Disease Control and Prevention
1600 Clifton Road, Northeast
Atlanta, GA 30333
404-639-3311 or 1-800-311-3435
www.cdc.gov

Food and Nutrition Information Center
National Agricultural Library
10301 Baltimore Avenue, Room 105
Beltsville, MD 20705
301-504-5414
www.nal.usda.gov/fnic

Weight-control Information Network
1 WIN Way
Bethesda, MD 20892-3665
877-946-4627
www.win.niddk.nih.gov/index.htm

National Institutes of Health
9000 Rockville Pike
Bethesda, MD 20892
301-496-4000
www.nih.gov

U.S. Food and Drug Administration
Office of Consumer Affairs, HFE 1
Room 16-85
5600 Fishers Lane
Rockville, MD 20857-0001
301-443-1726 or 1-800-463-6332
www.fda.gov

Grass-Fed Meat and Dairy Products

Peaceful Pastures
69 Cowan Valley Lane
Hickman, TN 38567
615-429-6806
www.peacefulpastures.com

Eat Wild (The Store for Healthy Living)
P.O. Box 7321
2401 North Cedar Street
Tacoma, WA 98406
1-866-453-8489
www.eatwild.com

Herbal Cleansing Products

Renew Life Formulas
2076 Sunnydale Boulevard
Clearwater, FL 33765
1-866-450-1787
www.renewlife.com

Hemorrhoid Treatment

Pilex®
202 Mirasol Way
Monterey, CA 93940-7639
831-333-0183
www.varicose.com

Laboratory Testing

Doctor's Data
(nutritional, gastrointestinal, immunology,
environmental screening)
3755 Illinois Avenue
St. Charles, IL 60174-2420
1-800-323-2784
www.doctorsdata.com

Genova Diagnostics
(endocrinology, gastrointestinal, immunology,
nutritional, metabolic testing)
63 Zillicoa Street
Asheville, NC 28801
828-253-0621
www.gdx.net

Mail-Order Organic Foods

Diamond Organics
1272 Highway 1
Moss Landing, CA 95039
1-888-ORGANIC (674-2642)
www.diamondorganics.com

Oraganics
419 68th Street
Brooklyn, NY 11220
1-800-991-8871
www.oraganic.com

Organic Provisions
P.O. Box 756
Richboro, PA 18954-0756
1-800-490-0044 or 215-674-2217
www.orgfood.com

Milk Products (Organic)

Organic Valley Family of Farms
CROPP Cooperative
1 Organic Way
LaFarge, WI 54639
1-888-444-6455
www.organicvalley.coop

Stonyfield Farm
10 Burton Drive
Londonderry, NH 03053
1-800-PRO-COWS (776-2697)
www.stonyfield.com

Nutrition

Price-Pottenger Nutrition Foundation
7890 Broadway
Lemon Grove, CA 91945
1-800-366-3748
www.price-pottenger.org

The Weston A. Price Foundation
PMB 106-380
4200 Wisconsin Avenue, NW
Washington, DC 20016
202-363-4394
www.westonaprice.org

Nuts and Seed Butters

Maranatha Nut Butters Mail Order
c/o WorldPantry.com
601 22nd Street
San Francisco, CA 94107
1-866-972-6879 or 415-401-0080
www.worldpantry.com

Once Again Nut Butter
12 South State Street
P.O. Box 429
Nunda, NY 14517-0429
1-888-800-8075
www.onceagainnutbutter.com

Oils (Organic Flax and Fish)

Foods Alive (liquid flax oil)
4840 County Road #4
Waterloo, IN 46793-9770
260-488-4497
www.foodsalive.com

Renew Life Formulas (fish oil capsules and flax oil capsules)
2076 Sunnydale Boulevard
Clearwater, FL 33765
1-866-450-1787
www.renewlife.com

Professional Organizations and Consumer Groups

American Diabetes Association
1701 North Beauregard Street
Alexandria, VA 22311
1-800-DIABETES (342-2383)
www.diabetes.org

American Obesity Association
1250 24th Street NW, Suite 300
Washington, DC 20037
202-776-7711
www.obesity.org

Center for Science in the Public Interest
1875 Connecticut Avenue NW, Suite 300
Washington, DC 20009
202-332-9110
www.cspinet.org

Consumers' Union
www.consumersunion.org

International Food Information Council Foundation
1100 Connecticut Avenue NW, Suite 430
Washington, DC 20036
202-296-6540
www.ific.org

Shape Up America!
www.shapeup.org

Free-Range Eggs

Pete and Gerry's Organic Eggs
140 Buffum Road
Monroe, NH 03771
1-800-GET-EGGS
www.peteandgerrys.com

Sauna (Infrared)

Renew Life Formulas
198 Alternate 19 North
Palm Harbor, FL 34683
1-866-450-1787
www.renewlife.com

Seagrass Meditation Chair

Santosha.com
1-888-288-9642
www.santosha.com

Weight Loss Support

Overeaters Anonymous
P.O. Box 44020
Rio Rancho, NM 87174-4020
505-891-2664
www.oa.org

NOTES

Introduction

1. American Obesity Association. For more information, visit www.obesity.org.

2. Judy Putnam, "U.S. Food Supply Providing More Food and Calories," *Food Review,* September—December 1999, www.findarticles.com/p/articles/mi_m3765/is_3_22/ai_61200979 (accessed November 10, 2006).

Chapter 1

1. Did You Know official Web site, www.didyouknow.cd/fastfacts/food.htm (accessed November 18, 2006).

2. For an in-depth look at any disease or condition, including statistics and general information, refer to the National Center for Health Statistics' official Web site at www.cdc.gov/nchs/htm. The NCHS is part of the U.S. government's Centers for Disease Control and Prevention (CDC). Its "Health Topics A to Z" is an invaluable source for data and information.

Chapter 2

1. M.A. Alfieri, J. Pomerleau, D.M. Grace, and L. Anderson. "Fiber Intake of Normal Weight, Moderately Obese and Severely Obese Subjects." *Obesity Research* 3:541–547 (1995).

2. I. Bourdon et al. "Postprandial Lipid, Glucose, Insulin, and Cholecystokinin Responses in Men Fed Barley Pasta Enriched with Beta-glucan." *American Journal of Clinical Nutrition* 69(1):55–63 (1969). The women in the study were split into three groups and fed three different breakfast meals. One meal was low-fiber/low-fat, another was high-fiber/low-fat, and the third was low-fiber/high-fat. Each of their CCK levels were measured before, during, and after their meals. Those who ate the high-fat and high-fiber meals reported greater feelings of fullness and their tests showed significantly higher levels of CCK in their blood than in those who ate the low-fat, low-fiber meals. Barbara Schneeman, a University of Califorina at Davis nutrition professor who led the study, said, "These results indicate that the addition of fiber to a meal can increase a person's feeling of being full. It appears this is due not only to fiber creating a greater volume of food in the gastrointestinal tract, but also to fiber promoting the release of cholecystokinin."

3. P.D. Cani, E. Joly, Y. Horsmans, and N.M. Delzenne. "Oligofructose Promotes Satiety in Healthy Human: A Pilot Study." *European Journal of Clinical Nutrition* 60(5):567–72 (2006).

4. K.R. Niness. "Inulin and Oligofructose: What Are They?" *Journal of Nutrition* 129(7 Suppl): 1402S—6S (1999).

5. A.F. Heini et al. "Effect of Hydrolyzed Guar Fiber on Fasting and Postprandial Satiety and Satiety Hormones: A Double-blind, Placebo-controlled Trial During Controlled Weight Loss." *International Journal of Obesity and Related Metabolic Disorders* 22(9):906–9 (1998). In this study, researchers from the Department of Nutrition at the University of Alabama studied the relationship of hydrolyzed guar gum supplementation (a type of fiber) and the cholecystokinin response over five weeks in twenty-five obese but otherwise healthy women. They were given

a reduced-calorie diet, and either a 20-gram fiber supplement (guar gum) or a placebo with their meals. Blood tests showed that after meals in which the fiber supplement was taken, cholecystokinin levels were at overall higher levels.

6. Audrey Eyton, *The F-Plan Diet* (New York: Crown, 1982), p. 18.

7. Mediterrasian's official Web site, www.mediterrasian.com/Fiber.htm (accessed November 2, 2005). See also the following study for more: D. Rigaud et al. "Effects of a Moderate Dietary Fibre Supplement on Hunger Rating, Energy Input and Faecal Energy Output in Young, Healthy Volunteers. A Randomized, Double-blind, Cross-over Trial." *International Journal of Obesity* 11 Suppl 1:73–8 (1987). This study found the same effect. Twenty young healthy volunteers of normal body weight, with a mean body mass index of 20.9, received a dietary fiber supplement of 7.3 grams per day in a randomized double-blind cross-over study. Those that received the fiber supplement, as compared to placebo, resulted in a significantly higher fecal energy (calorie) excretion. The study also found that moderate dietary fiber supplementation increased fecal energy excretion while simultaneously decreasing hunger.

8. E. Wisker, A. Maltz, and W. Feldheim. "Metabolizable Energy of Diets Low or High in Dietary Fiber from Cereals When Eaten by Humans." *Journal of Nutrition* 118(8):945–52 (1988).

9. S.J. Fairweather-Tait and A.J. Wright. "The Effect of 'Fibre-filler' (F-Plan Diet) on Iron, Zinc, and Calcium Absorption in Rats." *British Journal of Nutrition* 54(3):585–92 (1985).

10. *Journal of Nutrition*'s official Web site, http://jn.nutrition.org; in particular, http://jn.nutrition .org/cgi/reprint/130/2/272S.pdf (accessed December 15, 2005), "Symposium: Dietary Composition and Obesity: Do We Need to Look Beyond Dietary Fat?" by Britt Burton-Freeman; published by the American Society for Nutritional Sciences.

11. Ibid.

12. Ibid.

13. Studies also confirm the relationship between satiety and a particular volume of food. See www.aicr.org/pressrelease.lasso?index=1810 (accessed December 17, 2005).

14. Robert C. Atkins, M.D., *Dr. Atkins' New Diet Revolution* (New York: Avon Books, 2002), p. 49.

15. Ibid.

16. A.D. Liese et al. "Dietary Glycemic Index and Glycemic Load, Carbohydrate and Fiber Intake, and Measures of Insulin Sensitivity, Secretion, and Adiposity in the Insulin Resistance Atherosclerosis Study." *Diabetes Care* 28(12):2832–38 (2005). This study concluded that fiber was positively associated with insulin sensitivity. Refer also to C. Lau et al. "Dietary Glycemic Index, Glycemic Load, Fiber, Simple Sugars, and Insulin Resistance: The Inter99 Study." *Diabetes Care* 28(6):1397–403 (2005). In this other study, researchers examined cross-sectional associations between carbohydrate-related dietary factors and an estimate of insulin resistance in 5,675 subjects. They found that the intake of dietary fiber was inversely associated with the probability of having insulin resistance.

Chapter 3

1. The information regarding health benefits of soluble and insoluble fiber derive from Phyllis A. Balch, CNC, and James F. Balch, MD, *Prescription for Nutritional Healing,* 3rd ed. (New York: Penguin Putnam, 2000).

2. Top Cultures' informational site "Phytochemicals" at http://www.phytochemicals.info/.

3. B.J. Rolls, J.A. Ello-Martin, and B.C. Tohill. "What Can Intervention Studies Tell Us About the Relationship Between Fruit and Vegetable Consumption and Weight Management?" *Nutritional Reviews* 62(1):1–17 (2004).

4. The University of Miami's Miller School of Medicine's official Web site, "Medical Glossary," www.med.miami.edu/glossary/art.asp?articlekey=362 (accessed January 4, 2006).

Chapter 4

1. Barbara Ravage, *K.I.S.S. Guide to Weight Loss* (New York: Dorling Kindersley, 2001), p. 94.

2. Ibid., p. 96.

Chapter 5

1. A. Ascherio et al. "Trans-fatty Acids Intake and Risk of Myocardial Infarction." *Circulation* 89(1):94–101 (1994). Alice Lichtenstein, D.Sc., a professor of nutrition at Tufts University in Boston, has participated in several studies looking at the effects trans fats have on the body. One such study: J.F. Mauger et al. "Effect of Different Forms of Dietary Hydrogenated Fats on LDL Particle Size." *American Journal of Clinical Nutrition* 78(3):370–5 (2003).

2. A.M. Salter and D.A. White. "Effects of Dietary Fat on Cholesterol Metabolism: Regulation of Plasma LDL Concentrations." *Nutrition Research Reviews* 9:241–257 (1996). E. Lopez-Garcia et al. "Consumption of Trans Fatty Acids Is Related to Plasma Biomarkers of Inflammation and Endothelial Dysfunction." *Journal of Nutrition* 135(3):562–6 (2005).

3. F.F. Samaha. "Effect of Very High-fat Diets on Body Weight, Lipoproteins, and Glycemic Status in the Obese." *Curr Atheroscler Rep.* 7(6):412–20 (2005).

4. C.D. Gardner et al. "The Effect of a Plant-based Diet on Plasma Lipids in Hypercholesterolemic Adults: A Randomized Trial." *Annals of Internal Medicine* 142(9):725–33 (2005).

5. F.M. Sacks and H. Campos. "Polyunsaturated Fatty Acids, Inflammation, and Cardiovascular Disease: Time to Widen Our View of the Mechanisms." *Journal of Clinical Endocrinology and Metabolism* 91(2):398–400 (2006).

6. G.L. Khor. "Dietary Fat Quality: A Nutritional Epidemiologist's View." *Asia Pacific Journal of Clinical Nutrition* 13 (Suppl):S22 (2004).

7. "Dietary Supplementation with n-3 Polyunsaturated Fatty Acids and Vitamin E after Myocardial Infarction: Results of the GISSI-Prevenzione Trial." Gruppo Italiano per lo Studio della Sopravvivenza nell'Infarto miocardico. *Lance* 354(9177):447–55 (1999).

8. M.V. Chakravarthy et al. "'New' Hepatic Fat Activates PPARalpha to Maintain Glucose, Lipid, and Cholesterol Homeostasis." *Cell Metabolism* 1(5):309–22 (2005).

9. W.E. Lands. "Dietary Fat and Health: The Evidence and the Politics of Prevention: Careful Use of Dietary Fats Can Improve Life and Prevent Disease." *Annals of the New York Academy of Sciences* 1055:179–92 (2005).

10. B.V. Howard et al. "Low-fat Dietary Pattern and Risk of Cardiovascular Disease: The Women's Health Initiative Randomized Controlled Dietary Modification Trial." *Journal of the American Medical Association* 295(6):655–66 (2006).

11. For more about the benefits of coconut oil, refer to the following sources: I.A. Prior, F. Davidson et al. "Cholesterol, Coconuts, and Diet on Polynesian Atolls: A Natural Experiment: the Pukapuka and Tokelau Island Studies." *American Journal of Clinical Nutrition* 34(8):1552–61 (1981). S. Sircar and U. Kansra. "Choice of Cooking Oils—Myths and Realities." *Journal of the Indian Medical Association* 96(10):304–7 (1998). G.L. Blackburn et al. "A Reevaluation of Coconut Oil's Effect on Serum Cholesterol and Atherogenesis." *Journal of the Philippine Medical Association* 65:144–152 (1989). L.A. Cohen et al. "Dietary Fat and Mammary Cancer. I. Promoting Effects of Different Dietary Fats on N-nitrosomethylurea-induced Rat Mammary Tumorigenesis." *Journal of the National Cancer Institute* 77:33 (1986). L.A. Cohen et al. "Dietary Fat and Mammary Cancer. II. Modulation of Serum and Tumor Lipid Composition and Tumor Prostaglandins by Different Dietary Fats: Association with Tumor Incidence Patterns." *Journal of the National Cancer Institute* 77:43 (1986). Mary G. Enig, Ph.D. "Health and Nutritional Benefits from Coconut Oil: An Important Functional Food for the 21st Century." Presented at the AVOC Lauric Oils Symposium, Ho Chi Min City, Vietnam, April 25, 1996.

12. Dr. Joseph Mercola's official Web site, www.mercola.com/fcgi/pf/2005/jun/23/pasteurized_milk.htm (accessed January 5, 2006; page now discontinued). Analysis of data collected from more than 12,000 children between the ages of nine and fourteen, done over a twelve-month period to try to establish links between milk consumption and weight, found the following: The more milk children drank, the faster they gained weight; children who drank more than three 8-ounce servings of milk a day put on the most weight; the link held even though most of the children were drinking low-fat milk.

13. J.H. Lavin, S.J. French, and R.W. Read. "The Effect of Sucrose—and Aspartame-sweetened Drinks on Energy Intake, Hunger and Food Choice of Female, Moderately Restrained Eaters." *International Journal of Obesity and Related Metabolic Disorders* 21(1):37–42 (1997). T.L. Davidson and S.E. Swithers. "A Pavlovian Approach to the Problem of Obesity." *International Journal of Obesity and Related Metabolic Disorders* 28(7):933–35 (2004).

14. The following sites were accessed to obtain these statistics: www.sciencedaily.com/print.php?url=/releases/2005/05/050527111920.htm (accessed October 10, 2006; page now discontinued); http//www.mercola.com/2005/jun/14/calories_America.htm (accessed October 10, 2006). In addition: Daniel DeNoon, "Drink More Diet Soda, Gain More Weight?" http://my.webmd.com/content/article/107/108476.thm?src=rss_cbsnews (accessed November 18, 2006). As noted in DeNoon's article, data collected over an eight-year period of time by

researchers at the Texas Health Science Center in San Antonio, Texas, indicates that those who consume diet soft drinks have the following increase in risk for becoming overweight or obese:

36.5 percent for up to one can each day

37.5 percent for one can each day

54.5 percent for one to two cans each day

57.1 percent for more than two cans each day

The head researcher in this study points to another recent study in which rat pups fed artificial sweeteners craved more calories than animals fed real sugar.

15. T.A. Nicklas, T. Baranowski, K.W. Cullen, and G. Berenson. "Eating Patterns, Dietary Quality and Obesity." *Journal of the American College of Nutrition* 20:599–608 (2001).

Chapter 7

1. M.A. Pereira et al. "Effects of a Low-glycemic Load Diet on Resting Energy Expenditure and Heart Disease Risk Factors During Weight Loss." *Journal of the American Medical Association* 292(20):2482–90 (2004).

2. The following batches of studies point to the benefits found in banaba extract, conjugated linoleic acid (CLA), and medium chain triglycerides (MCT) respectively: H. Hong and W. Jai Maeng. "Effects of Malted Barley Extract and Banaba Extract on Blood Glucose Levels in Genetically Diabetic Mice." *Journal of Medicinal Food* 7(4):487–90 (2004). M.Y. Park, K.S. Lee, and M.K. Sung. "Effects of Dietary Mulberry, Korean Red Ginseng, and Banaba on Glucose Homeostasis in Relation to PPAR-alpha, PPAR-gamma, and LPL mRNA Expressions." *Life Sciences* 77(26):3344–54 (2005). Epub June 23, 2005.

U. Riserus, L. Berglund, and B. Vessby. "Conjugated Linoleic Acid (CLA) Reduced Abdominal Adipose Tissue in Obese Middle-aged Men with Signs of the Metabolic Syndrome: A Randomised Controlled Trial." *International Journal of Obesity and Related Metabolic Disorders* 25(8):1129–35 (2001). M.M. Kamphuis, M.P. Lejeune, W.H. Saris, and M.S. Westerterp-Plantenga. "The Effect of Conjugated Linoleic Acid Supplementation After Weight Loss on Body Weight Regain, Body Composition, and Resting Metabolic Rate in Overweight Subjects." *International Journal of Obesity and Related Metabolic Disorders* 27(7):840–7 (2003). J.M. Gaullier et al. "Conjugated Linoleic Acid Supplementation for 1 Year Reduces Body Fat Mass in Healthy Overweight Humans." *American Journal of Clinical Nutrition* 79(6):1118–25 (2004).

M.P. St-Onge, R. Ross, W.D. Parsons, and P.J. Jones. "Medium-chain Triglycerides Increase Energy Expenditure and Decrease Adiposity in Overweight Men." *Obesity Research* 11(3):395–402 (2003). A.A. Papamandjaris, M.D. White, M. Raeini-Sarjaz, P.J. Jones. "Endogenous Fat Oxidation During Medium Chain versus Long Chain Triglyceride Feeding in Healthy Women." *International Journal of Obesity and Related Metabolic Disorders* 24(9):1158–66 (2000).

3. K. Spiegel et al. "Leptin Levels Are Dependent on Sleep Duration: Relationships with Sympathovagal Balance, Carbohydrate Regulation, Cortisol, and Thyrotropin." *Journal of Clinical*

Endocrinology and Metabolism 89(11):5762–71 (2004). S. Taheri et al. "Short Sleep Duration Is Associated with Reduced Leptin, Elevated Ghrelin, and Increased Body Mass Index." *Public Library of Science Medicine* 1(3):e62 (2004). Epub December 7, 2004.

Chapter 9

1. Ecological Rights Foundation Public Information Web site, "Toxins in Our Environment" (accessed November 2, 2006).

2. P. Imbeault et al. "Weight Loss-induced in Plasma Pollutant Is Associated with Reduced Skeletal Muscle Oxidative Capacity." *American Journal of Physiology—Endocrinology and Metabolism* 282(3):E574–79 (2002).

3. Evironmental Working Group, "Body Burden: The Pollution in People," http://www.ewg/reports/bodyburden1/es.php (accessed November 2, 2006).

4. Department of Health and Human Services, Centers for Disease Control and Prevention, official Web site at www.cdc.gov; "Exposure Report" from July 21, 2005; http://www.cdc.gov/exposurereport (accessed November 8, 2006).

5. Brenda Watson, C.T., and Leonard Smith, M.D., "Probiotics and the Anti-Aging Revolution," in J. Ghen Mitchell et al., ed. *The Advanced Guide to Longevity Medicine.* (Mitchell J. Ghen, D.O., Ph.D., 2001), 203–209.

6. M.D. Anway, A.S. Cupp, M. Uzumcu, and M.K. Skinner. "Epigenetic Transgenerational Actions of Endocrine Disruptors and Male Fertility." *Science* 308(5727):1466–9 (2005). J. Kaiser. "Developmental Biology. Endocrine Disrupters Trigger Fertility Problems in Multiple Generations." *Science* 308(5727):1391–92 (2005).

7. P. Imbeault et al. "Weight Loss-induced in Plasma Pollutant Is Associated with Reduced Skeletal Muscle Oxidative Capacity." *American Journal of Physiology—Endocrinology and Metabolism* 282(3):E574–79 (2002).

8. Pelletier et al., "Associations Between Weight-loss-induced Changes in Plasma Organochlorine Concentrations, Serum T3 Concentration, and Resting Metabolic Rate." *Toxicological Sciences,* 67 (2002): 46–51.

9. P. Imbeault. "Weight Loss-induced in Plasma Pollutant Is Associated with Reduced Skeletal Muscle Oxidative Capacity." *American Journal of Physiology—Endocrinology and Metabolism* 282(3):E574–79 (2002).

10. Mark Hyman, M.D., *Ultra-Metabolism* (New York: Scribner, 2006), p. 195.

11. Environmental Working Group, "Beauty Secrets: Executive Summary," http://www.ewg.org/reports/bearutysecrets/execsumm.html (accessed November 8, 2006).

12. Dr. Bernard Jensen, *Dr. Jensen's Guide to Diet and Detoxification: Healthy Secrets from Around the World* (Lincolnwood, Ill.: Keats, 2000), p. 75.

Chapter 10

1. A. Belluzzi. "Effect of an Enteric-coated Fish-oil Preparation on Relapses in Crohn's Disease." *New England Journal of Medicine* 334(24):1557–60 (1996).

Chapter 11

1. L.J. Cheskin. "Mechanisms of Constipation in Older Persons and Effects of Fiber Compared with Placebo." *Journal of the American Geriatric Society* 43(6):666–9 (1995).

2. W.H. Aldoori et al. "A Prospective Study of Dietary Fiber Types and Symptomatic Diverticular Disease in Men." *Journal of Nutrition* 128(4):714–9 (1998). W.H. Aldoori et al. "A Prospective Study of Diet and the Risk of Symptomatic Diverticular Disease in Men." *American Journal of Clinical Nutrition* 60(5):757–64 (1994).

3. C.J. Tsai, M.F. Leitzmann, W.C. Willett, and E.L. Giovannucci. "Long-term Intake of Dietary Fiber and Decreased Risk of Cholecystectomy in Women." *American Journal of Gastroenterology* 99(7):1364–70 (2004).

4. H.B. El-Serag, J.A. Satia, and L. Rabeneck. "Dietary Intake and the Risk of Gastro-oesophageal Reflux Disease: a Cross Sectional Study in Volunteers." *Gut* 54(1):11–17(2005).

5. M.A. Pereira, E. O'Reilly, K. Augustsson et al. "Dietary Fiber and Risk of Coronary Heart Disease." *Archives of Internal Medicine* 164:370–6 (2004). The Harvard scientists concluded, "our results suggest that dietary fiber intake during adulthood is inversely associated with coronary heart disease (CHD) risk. . . . The recommendations to consume a diet that includes an abundance of fiber-rich foods to prevent CHD are based on a wealth of consistent scientific evidence."

6. L. A. Bazzano et al. "Dietary Fiber Intake and Reduced Risk of Coronary Heart Disease in US Men and Women: The National Health and Nutrition Examination Survey I Epidemiologic Follow-up Study." *Archives of Internal Medicine* 163:1897–1904 (2003).

7. L.A. Bazzano et al. "Fruit and Vegetable Intake and Risk of Cardiovascular Disease in US Adults: The First National Health and Nutrition Examination Survey Epidemiologic Follow-up Study." *American Journal of Clinical Nutrition* 76(1):93–99 (2002).

8. The National Institutes of Health, National Library of Medicine's official Web site, Medline Plus, http://www.nlm.nih.gov/medlineplus/print/new/fullstory_26677.html (accessed March 28, 2006).

9. American Heart Association Meeting report, April 30, 2005, "Fiber Supplements May Lower Cardiovascular Risk in Type 2 Diabetics."

10. William Davis, M.D., *Track Your Plaque: The Only Heart Disease Prevention Program That Shows How to Use the New Heart Scans to Detect, Track, and Control Coronary Plaque* (iUniverse, 2004).

11. M.A. Pereira, E. O'Reilly, K. Augustsson et al. "Dietary Fiber and Risk of Coronary Heart Disease." *Archives of Internal Medicine* 164:370–76 (2004).

12. P.M. Kearney et al. "Global Burden of Hypertension: Analysis of Worldwide Data." *Lancet* 365(9455):217–23 (2005).

13. E. Saltzman et al. "An Oat-containing Hypocaloric Diet Reduces Systolic Blood Pressure and Improves Lipid Profile Beyond Effects of Weight Loss in Men and Women."*Journal of Nutrition* 131(5):1465–70 (2001).

14. FDA Consumer, July–August 1997, "Bulking Up Fiber's Healthful Reputation," http://seniorhealth.about.com/cs/nutrition/a/diet_fiber_p.htm, referencing a December 1996 study, "Intake of Dietary Fiber and Risk of Coronary Heart Disease in a Cohort of Finnish Men," published in *Circulation* 94:2720–27 (1996). E.B. Rimm et al. "Vegetable, Fruit, and Cereal Fiber Intake and Risk of Coronary Heart Disease Among Men." *Journal of the American Medical Association* 275(6):447–51 (1996).

15. Ibid.

16. Jennifer Warner, "Fiber May Cut Some Risks of Secondhand Smoke," article posted September 1, 2005 on WebMD's official Web site, http://my.webmd.com/content/Article/111/109885.htm?z=1728_00000_1000_tn_09 (accessed November 16, 2006). Original source: G.L. David et al. "Childhood Exposure to Environmental Tobacco Smoke and Chronic Respiratory Symptoms in Non-smoking Adults: The Singapore Chinese Health Study." *Thorax* 60(12):1052–58 (2005). Epub August 30, 2005.

17. T. Terashima et al. "The Fusion of Bone-marrow-derived Proinsulin-expressing Cells with Nerve Cells Underlies Diabetic Neuropathy." *Proceedings of the National Academy of Science of the U.S.A.* 102(35):12525–30 (2005). Epub August 22, 2005.

18. "Dietary Patterns and the Risk for Type 2 Diabetes in U.S. Men." *Annals of Internal Medicine* 136(3):I30 (2002).

19. T.T. Fung et al. "Whole-grain Intake and the Risk of Type 2 diabetes: A Prospective Study in Men." *American Journal of Clinical Nutrition* 76(3):535–40 (2002).

20. M. Uusitupa. "Lifestyles Matter in the Prevention of Type 2 Diabetes." *Diabetes Care* 25(9):1650–51 (2002).

21. For a complete review of this experiment, as well as other supporting studies, refer to HCF Nutrition Foundation's official Web site at www.hcfnutrition.org, "Obesity," and "Fiber and Obesity."

22. Ibid.

23. Studies that point to fiber's positive effect on blood sugar balance are numerous. I can't possibly list all the studies that show how amazing fiber is as a natural balancer of blood sugar. For those who suffer from diabetes, adding more fiber can help keep insulin levels more stable; this stability in turn helps prevent the accumulation of fat. A study at the University of Texas Southwestern Medical Center at Dallas, for example, found that eating large amounts of fiber in foods like okra, beans, and sweet potatoes significantly lowers blood sugar in people with diabetes. People consuming 50 grams of fiber a day lowered their blood sugar by 10 percent. In

addition, insulin levels dropped and LDL (bad cholesterol) also went down. The foods used in this study included oranges, grapefruit, cantaloupe, papayas, raisins, winter and zucchini squash, granola, and oat bran. The Texas researchers concluded that "diet is the mainstay of diabetes treatment but is often neglected. The study supports the view that diet can improve glucose and lipid levels and thus reduce the risk of long-term diabetic complications." (Aside from the large amounts of fiber, the diets used in the study incorporated the Mediterranean diet, which focuses on fruits and vegetables, whole grains and olive oil.) For more information, refer to the study: M. Chandalia et al. "Beneficial Effects of High Dietary Fiber Intake in Patients with Type 2 Diabetes Mellitus." *New England Journal of Medicine* 342(19):1392–98 (2000).

24. C.K. Roberts. "Effect of a Diet and Exercise Intervention on Oxidative Stress, Inflammation and Monocyte Adhesion in Diabetic Men." *Diabetes Research and Clinical Practice* 73(3):249–59 (2006). Epub April 17 2006. Drs. James Barnard and Christian Roberts of UCLA have been at the forefront of diabetes research. In a recent investigation, they followed thirteen diabetic men at the Pritikin Longevity Center for three weeks, finding that the Pritikin high-fiber, high-carb diet and daily exercise not only helped the men lose weight and improve cholesterol levels but also decreased blood sugar levels by 20 percent and insulin levels by 30 percent. What's more, by the end of their three-week program, six of the thirteen men had controlled their blood sugar levels so well that "they were not classified as diabetic." The men finished the experiment completely free of their diabetic medications, "and others had their medication dosages reduced."

25. L.E. Kelemen et al. "Vegetables, Fruit, and Antioxidant-related Nutrients and Risk of Non-Hodgkin Lymphoma: A National Cancer Institute-Surveillance, Epidemiology, and End Results Population-based Case-control Study." *American Journal of Clinical Nutrition* 83(6):1401–10 (2006).

26. G. Danaei et al. "Causes of Cancer in the World: Comparative Risk Assessment of Nine Behavioural and Environmental Risk Factors." *Lancet* 366(9499):1784–93 (2005).

27. T. Pischon et al. "Body Size and Risk of Colon and Rectal Cancer in the European Prospective Investigation into Cancer and Nutrition (EPIC)." *Journal of the National Cancer Institute* 98(13):920–31 (2006). Scientists disagree on the precise role of fiber in lowering the risk of colon cancer, although no one argues that it isn't helpful. "Results from one of the largest studies ever conducted into the link between diet and cancer—the EPIC (European Prospective Investigation of Cancer and Nutrition) Study—involving more than 400,000 people from nine countries for nearly five years, found that the people eating the most fiber had a 40 percent lower risk of colon cancer than those people eating the least." This effect is thought to result from the increased movement of potentially carcinogenic substances through the GI tract. But U.S. scientists, analyzing studies of fiber's effects on colon cancer, cast doubt on this preventive benefit. Who's right? The European scientists argue that the American researchers at Harvard University have not looked at the latest data, which shows that fiber does protect the colon. Meanwhile, the Americans admit that "although high dietary fiber intake may not have a major effect on the risk of colorectal (bowel) cancer, a diet high in dietary fiber from whole plant foods can be advised because this has been related to lower risks of other chronic conditions such as heart disease and diabetes." Translation: this study didn't find an effect on colon cancer, as the Europeans

did, but fiber is still very beneficial. For more, see the following article: J.A. Baron. "Dietary Fiber and Colorectal Cancer: An Ongoing Saga." *Journal of the American Medical Association* 294(22):2904–6 (2005).

28. J.M. Chan, F. Wang, and E.A. Holly. "Vegetable and Fruit Intake and Pancreatic Cancer in a Population-based Case-control Study in the San Francisco Bay Area." *Cancer Epidemiological Biomarkers Prevention* (9):2093–7 (2005).

29. M. Kivipelto et al. "Obesity and Vascular Risk Factors at Midlife and the Risk of Dementia and Alzheimer Disease." *Archives of Neurology 62*:1556–60 (2005).

Chapter 12

1. H.J. Heo et al. "Apple Phenolics Protect in Vitro Oxidative Stress-induced Neuronal Cell Death." *Journal of Food Science* 69(9):S357–60. "The studies show that additional apple consumption may not only help reduce the risk of cancer, as previous studies have shown, but also that an apple a day may supply major bioactive compounds, which may play an important role in reducing the risk of neurodegenerative disorders," notes Chang Y. Lee, PhD, a professor of food science at Cornell.

Dr. Lee's laboratory research found that the higher the concentration of apple phenolic extract, the more protection nerves enjoyed against oxidative stress. "What we found was that the apple phenolics, which are naturally occurring antioxidants found in fresh apples, can protect nerve cells from neurotoxicity induced by oxidative stress," Dr. Lee states. According to these studies, quercetin defends nerve cells against oxidative damage even more effectively than vitamin C. Besides apples, quercetin is abundant in berries and onions. Dr. Lee has also found that the phytonutrients in apples are potentially protective against colon and liver cancer.

2. J. Limpens et al. "Combined Lycopene and Vitamin E Treatment Suppresses the Growth of PC-346C Human Prostate Cancer Cells in Nude Mice." *Journal of Nutrition* 136(5):1287–93 (2006). The researchers conclude that "we would certainly recommend that all men regularly eat lycopene and vitamin E–rich foods: for example, all kinds of processed tomato products, papayas, pink grapefruit and watermelon, wheat germs, whole grains, mangoes, leafy green vegetables, nuts, and olive oils."

3. J.H. Cohen, A.R. Kristal, and J.L. Stanford. "Fruit and Vegetable Intakes and Prostate Cancer Risk." *Journal of the National Cancer Institute* 92(1):61–8 (2000). "The bottom line is that if you eat a lot of vegetables, you can cut your risk of prostate cancer by about 45 percent," says researcher Alan Kristal, PhD. "And, if some of those vegetables are from the cruciferous family, like broccoli and cabbage, you may reduce your risk even further."

4. T.O. Khor et al. "Combined Inhibitory Effects of Curcumin and Phenethyl Isothiocyanate on the Growth of Human PC-3 Prostate Xenografts in Immunodeficient Mice." *Cancer Research* 66(2):61321 (2006).

5. M. Green et al. "Diallyl Sulfide Inhibits Diethylstilbesterol-induced DNA Adducts in the Breast of Female ACI Rats." *Food and Chemical Toxicology* 43(9):1323–31 (2005). Epub April 14, 2005.

6. O.H. Franco et al. "The Polymeal: A More Natural, Safer, and Probably Tastier (Than the Polypill) Strategy to Reduce Cardiovascular Disease by More than 75%." *British Medical Journal* 329(7480):1447–50 (2004).

7. A. Davalos et al. "Red Grape Juice Polyphenols Alter Cholesterol Homeostasis and Increase LDL-receptor Activity in Human Cells in Vitro." *Journal of Nutrition* 136(7):1766–73 (2006).

8. M.B. Schabath et al. "Dietary Phytoestrogens and Lung Cancer Risk." *Journal of the American Medical Association* 294(12):1493–504 (2005).

Chapter 13

1. W.R. Lovallo et al. "Caffeine Stimulation of Cortisol Secretion Across the Waking Hours in Relation to Caffeine Intake Levels." *Psychosomatic Medicine* 67(5):734–39 (2005).

2. www.weight.com/Leptin.html (accessed November 15, 2006).

3. Dr. Joseph Mercola, *The No-Grain Diet* (NewYork: Dutton, 2003), p. 146.

4. Michael F. Roizen, M.D., and Mehmet C. Oz, M.D., *You: The Owner's Manual* (New York: HarperResource, 2005), p. 192.

5. R.H. Lustig. "Childhood Obesity: Behavioral Aberration or Biochemical Drive? Reinterpreting the First Law of Thermodynamics." *Nature Clinical Practice Endocrinology and Metabolism* 2(8):447–58 (2006).

6. J.D. Artiss et al. "The Effects of a New Soluble Dietary Fiber on Weight Gain and Selected Blood Parameters in Rats." *Metabolism* 55(2):195–202 (2006).

7. Ann Louise Gittleman, MS, CNS, *The Fat Flush Plan* (New York: McGraw-Hill, 2002), p. 25.

8. Ibid.

Chapter 14

1. All calorie counts for meals were calculated with the help of a nutritional analysis program. Because exact amounts will vary depending on how you measure and prepare your ingredients, view these calorie counts as estimates. Go to www.nutritiondata.com for further help in calculating calories if you choose to modify a recipe.

GENERAL INDEX

abdominal fat, 99, 162
abdominals, exercises for, 118, 124–25
acacia, 27, 146, 147
acetic acid, 129
acidity, 27
acid reflux, 152–53
activewear, 113
activity calories, 45
adaptogenic herbs, 178
adrenal burnout, 177
adrenal glands, 16, 144, 176, 177, 178
adrenocorticotrophic hormone
     (ACTH), 176, 177
advanced glycation end products
     (AGEs), 179
adzuki beans, 67
aerobic exercise, 89, 100–101, 125
aging, 31
Agriculture, U.S. Department of, 18
air conditioners, 133
alcohol, 74
alder buckthorn, 137
alkalinity, 27
allergies, 31, 74
allicin, 31
aloe, 137, 144
alpha linolenic acid (ALA), 57
alpha lipoic acid, 137
Alzheimer's disease, 31, 164
amaranth, 69
American Diabetes Association, 68
amino acids, 42, 51–52, 144, 145, 178
anaerobic exercise, 100
anasazi beans, 67
Anderson Cancer Center, 171
animals, grass-fed, 52
anthocyanin, 30
antioxidants, 30, 142, 167, 168
apoptosis, 170

appaloosa beans, 67
appetite control, 9, 10, 14
apples, 26, 63, 71, 72
apricots, 64
arachadonic acid, 52
arginine, 107
arterial nitric oxide synthetase (NOS),
     107
arteries, 155
arthritis, 31, 57, 98
ascorbic acid, 143
ascorbyl palmitate, 143
ashwaganda, 144, 178
aspartame, 68
atherosclerosis, 153, 155
autoimmune diseases, 31
avocados, 60

back exercises, 116, 118–19
back pain, 98
bacteria, 31
bakeries, 256, 267
bamboo leaf extract, 102
banaba, 99, 102, 143, 144, 184
bananas, 64, 71
barley, 26, 69
bars, high-fiber, 147
beans, 66–67, 267
   and cancer, 162
   dried, 27
   fiber in, 32, 67, 71
   overnight soaking of, 66
beets, 26, 65, 72
berries, 64, 72
beta-glucans, 25
biceps exercises, 117, 121
Bi Curls, 117, 121
Bifidobacteria bifidum, 129
bile, 17, 152, 156

RECIPE INDEX

ABOUT THE AUTHORS

Brenda Watson, C.N.C., is a bestselling author and one of the foremost dietary authorities in America today. She has gained national recognition with her televised PBS specials *Brenda Watson's H.O.P.E. Formula: The Ultimate Health Secret* and *Brenda Watson's The Fiber35 Diet: Nature's Weight Loss Secret.* She is also the author of the forthcoming *The Detox Prescription: Vibrant Health in 5 Easy Steps* (Free Press, 2008), which will also have a PBS special in March 2008. Ms. Watson has two grown children and currently lives in Florida with her husband, Stan, and their dogs.

Leonard Smith, M.D., is a renowned general gastrointestinal and vascular surgeon as well as an expert in nutrition and natural supplementation. He is a board-certified general surgeon and is currently a member of the volunteer faculty at the University of Miami Department of Surgery. Dr. Smith has been a surgeon in Florida for twenty-five years and resides there with his wife and two grown daughters.